The
Acute-Care
Nurse
Practitioner

The
Acute-Care Nurse Practitioner

A Transformational Journey

Judy Rashotte

AU PRESS

Published by AU Press, Athabasca University
1200, 10011 – 109 Street, Edmonton, AB T5J 3S8

ISBN 978-1-927356-26-5 (print) 978-1-927356-27-2 (PDF) 978-1-927356-28-9 (epub)

Cover and interior design by Natalie Olsen, Kisscut Design
Cover photography: taretz / photocase.com, Raffiella / photocase.com,
es.war.einmal.. / photocase.com, Eisenglimmer / photocase.com
Printed and bound in Canada by Marquis Book Printers

Library and Archives Canada Cataloguing in Publication
Rashotte, Judy, 1952–
The acute-care nurse practitioner : a transformational journey /
by Judy Rashotte.

Includes bibliographical references.
Issued also in electronic formats.
ISBN 978-1-927356-26-5

1. Nurse practitioners – Canada – Biography.
2. Nurse practitioners – Canada – Attitudes.
3. Nurse practitioners – Canada – Anecdotes.
4. Intensive care nursing – Canada – Anecdotes.
I. Title.

RT82.8.R38 2013   610.73092'271   C2012-905790-8

We acknowledge the financial support of the Government of Canada
through the Canada Book Fund (CBF) for our publishing activities.

Canada Council   Conseil des Arts
for the Arts   du Canada

Assistance provided by the Government of Alberta, Alberta Multimedia
Development Fund.

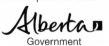

Government

Words mean more than we mean to express when we use them; so a whole book ought to mean a great deal more than the writer means. So, whatever good meanings are in the book, I'm very glad to accept as the meaning of the book.
— **Lewis Carroll**

Contents

List of Figures

Acknowledgements

To acute-care nurse practitioners who have inspired me and whose contributions formed the basis for this book.

To Louise Jensen, Wendy Austin, Brenda Cameron, and Karen Golden-Biddle for their expertise, respect, commitment, patience, and belief in my abilities.

To my sons, Peter and Joseph, and my husband, Barry, without whom I would not feel whole. Their unfailing love and support makes it possible for me to take my own journeys.

To Margot, my colleague and friend, whose positive spirit and wise counsel sustain me.

I gratefully acknowledge the financial support provided through the Izaak Walton Killam Memorial Scholarship, as well as additional funding in the form of awards, fellowships, studentships, and internships received throughout my studies from the Children's Hospital of Eastern Ontario, the Children's Hospital of Eastern Ontario Research Institute, the Canadian Nurses Foundation, the University of Alberta, the Canadian Association of Critical Care, and the Registered Nurses Association of Ontario, Nursing Leadership Network.

Introduction

In this book, I examine the experience of nurse practitioners (NPs) working in acute-care settings within tertiary-care institutions across Canada. The material for this book came from a study employing hermeneutic phenomenology, a research genre intended to construct a full interpretive description of a given human experience as we meet it in the world, to cause us to engage in reflection, and to challenge the way we have previously seen and understood the world. In this book I describe the different perspectives from which people view their reality as they undergo a transformational journey of becoming and being in the acute-care NP role. I also explore how they struggle to engage in a meaningful practice that fulfills what they desire as nurses, and examine how their journeys are promoted and hindered. A natural inclination is to assume that this book is intended only for NPs, particularly those working in acute-care settings. But this would be an erroneous assumption. We have all undergone transformational changes in our lives — moved away from home, become a nurse, physician, educator, administrator, spouse, or parent — all of which resulted in journeys that were fraught with complex emotions, thoughts, and actions. Therefore, parts of this book may resonate with many readers irrespective of their roles in the health care system. I also hope that the information in this book will help all of us who work alongside, receive care from, mentor, teach, or supervise NPs to better understand what is most common, most taken for granted, and what concerns us most about the lived experience of being an NP.

Much of this book is based on extensive interviews with acute-care NPs who perceive themselves as living professional lives and who have a sense of ordinary, daily routine. Yet in the ordinary activities of their day-to-day practice the extraordinary is made visible. Because of this extraordinary, complex, and multidimensional nature of the NPs' experiences, I make use of the works of poets, authors, and artists to construct a more animated and powerful description and interpretation of their journey. Furthermore, although I acknowledge that every individual's journey is unique, there are universal meanings that are more evocatively revealed in poetry, literature, or painting. Therefore my conversation with others, including other theorists and researchers, is an important part of this book, because "it is in this material that the human being can be found as *situated person*" (van Manen, 1997, p. 19), not only in this moment, but also through time.

The Research Journey

I understood from Beth's explanation to the mother that the baby was showing signs of a systemic infection and needed to start antibiotics right away. She was preparing to insert an intravenous catheter into one of the baby's central veins, which would be the best way to administer the medication over the next week or so. Beth was a neonatal nurse practitioner with five years of experience in this role. Her movements were methodical as she gathered the equipment from the shelves. She explained the procedure she was about to undertake with this sick infant in a soft, gentle voice, offered the mother the choice to wait outside the unit or to remain at the bedside, then situated the stool across from where she would be working, facilitating the mother's access to the proceedings. She gently positioned the baby, intermittently stroking his head and massaging his feet, and then, with the bedside nurse's assistance, she silently undertook the procedure with composure and self-assurance embedded within demonstrations of caring. Upon completion of the procedure, Beth cleared away the debris while the bedside nurse and mother resettled the baby. When the mother returned to the rocking chair by the bedside, Beth sat down beside her and I heard her ask the mother what was the most pressing concern she had at that moment. The mother was crying as she expressed her regret that the strides she had finally been able to make with her baby taking the breast would be halted, just another reason to feel like a failure as a mother. Beth gently took the mother's hands into hers and in a soft, tender voice she began to explore with her what it was like to be the mother of a sick premature infant.

Researchers are drawn to study that which has personal significance. I am not, nor have I ever been, a nurse practitioner (NP). However, in my previous nursing management role in a tertiary-care institution, I frequently heard physicians say to student NPs, "You need to think more like a physician." I heard student and novice NPs express regret about the decision to become an NP because they no longer felt like nurses and did not want to be physician replacements. Through their tears, they repeatedly asked, "Where is the nurse in what I do?" I was involved in administrative decisions that determined whether NPs or physicians would provide the medical care in areas that were experiencing resident shortages — decisions that focused entirely on discussions regarding cost-effectiveness and overlapping functionalities. Yet the above story of how the NP cared for a sick infant and his mother was not an isolated one. I had seen NPs massaging their patients' limbs before and after performing potentially painful procedures, and hugging fathers and mothers when they had just informed them that their child was dying.

I came to this study because I had found myself caught up short every time I witnessed these types of caring actions. Was it because they were incongruent with what I had heard and read about NPs? Had I been unduly influenced by the dominant discourses? Was what I had observed an aberration or had it not been given a voice? Was the way I viewed NPs working in hospital-based practices not so much about incongruence but more about incompleteness?

Background of the Study

Nurse practitioners are "registered nurses with additional educational preparation and experience who possess and demonstrate the competencies to autonomously diagnose, order, and interpret diagnostic tests, prescribe pharmaceuticals, and perform specific procedures within their legislated cope of practice" (Canadian Nurses Association [CNA], 2009, p. 1). The role was first introduced in the United States in the 1960s. In the 1970s, the concept of an expanded practice role for nurses gained momentum in Canada, and six Canadian universities offered programs to prepare NPs to provide primary health care, particularly in Canada's northern and rural communities (Patterson, 1997). Approximately 250 NPs educated in these programs between 1970 and 1983 filled the perceived health care gap created by physician shortages in the 1960s. The creation of the role, while at times controversial in terms of title and function, provided the nursing profession with an opportunity to expand its scope of practice and begin to demonstrate nursing's impact on the health status of Canadians.

Competition for patients occurred as the number of physicians increased in the late 1970s and early 1980s (Kaasalainen et al., 2010). This, combined with the absence of an effective payment structure and little public understanding of the NP role, resulted in the underutilization of these practitioners and a subsequent lack of practice opportunities, despite the Boudreau Committee's recommendation that the development of the NP role in primary health care be given a high priority (Boudreau, 1972). The NP educational initiative was withdrawn by the early 1980s; a lack of recognition of the nursing component within the NP role was a significant factor in closing NP programs. The result was a stigma that NPs were physician replacements, perpetuated in part by increasing resistance to the role from both the medical and nursing communities (Gortner, 1982; Rogers, 1975; Sandelowski, 2000), a resistance that continues in Canada thirty years later.

Then, in the late 1980s and early 1990s, the need for cost containment and efficiency resulted in demands that innovative approaches to Canadian health care delivery be quickly developed and initiated, causing a renewed interest in the role. Moreover, advances in technology, higher levels of acuity, and shortened hospital stays, combined with the downsizing of residency programs in teaching hospitals, resulted in increasingly fragmented care and shortages of in-hospital medical coverage for acutely ill patients (Barer and Stoddart, 1992a, 1992b, 1992c), all factors that have been cited as the impetus for the widespread introduction of acute-care NPs (Hravnak et al., 2009; Paes et al., 1989; Pringle, 2007). In 1988, the number of Canadian universities offering graduate-level nursing programs to prepare NPs for tertiary care began to increase (Canadian Institute of Health Information [CIHI], 2006; Canadian Nurse Practitioner Initiative

[CNPI], 2005). This number has continued to rise as a result of provincial funding and legislative initiatives (CIHI, 2010), demonstrating ongoing political and economic support.

All 13 provinces and territories in Canada have NP legislation and regulation. Ten of these jurisdictions recognize NPs working in hospital-based practices (CIHI, 2006; CNA, 2006; Health Professions Regulatory Advisory Council [HPRAC], 2007a, 2007b). In New Brunswick, the Northwest Territories, and Nunavut, only primary health care/family NPs are eligible for registration (HPRAC, 2007a, 2007b). *Nurse practitioner* is now a legislated protected title across Canada. The CNA, in partnership with the provincial nursing associations and regulatory colleges in Canada, developed entry-level competencies for all NPs, recognizing three streams of practice: family/all ages, adult, and child. NPs who had previously informally adopted the term *acute-care nurse practitioner*, such as graduates educated to work in NP roles in teaching hospitals, wrote certification exams for the first time in 2008.

Two types of discourse — instrumental and economic — have dominated the NP research (Rashotte, 2005). Instrumental discourse, which objectifies NPs in their role, has described, studied, and discussed their activities within an overarching framework of business, with the intention to build an adequate representation of the NP role. Researchers have analyzed and discussed the NP role in terms of NPs' demographics, educational preparation, geographic region of practice, years of employment, and type of employment setting (Hurlock-Chorostecki, van Soreren, and Goodwin, 2008; Sidani et al., 2000); position titles and reporting relationships (Centre for Nursing Studies, 2001); role clarity and role utilization (Donald et al., 2010); role classification, responsibilities, and functions (Kleinpell, 2002, 2005; Kleinpell et al., 2006); decision-making processes as compared to those of physicians (Carnevale, 2001; Offredy, 1998); and facilitators and barriers to implementing hospital-based NPs (Cummings, Fraser, and Tarlier, 2003; Kilpatrick et al., 2010; Reay, Golden-Biddle, and GermAnn, 2003, 2006; Roschkov et al., 2007; Schreiber et al., 2005; van Soeren and Micevski, 2001). Judging from the results of more than 30 years of research, the quality of care provided by NPs has equalled and, in some instances, exceeded that provided by physicians in the same practice, and has enhanced collaborative relationships with all members of the health care team (Carter and Chochinov, 2007; Hoffman et al., 2005; Mitchell-DiCenso et al., 1996; Russell, VorderBruegge, and Burns, 2002; Sidani et al., 2006). In addition, studies have confirmed that patients are accepting of and satisfied with NP services (Fanta et al., 2006; Sidani, 2008).

Many of the studies have been embedded in Hamric, Spross, and Hanson's (1996) framework for the advanced practice nurse centred on five domains of practice — expert clinician, consultant, educator, researcher, and leader/change agent — or on the Canadian Nurse Practitioner Core Competency Framework (CNPI, 2004). In Canada, NPs and clinical nurse specialists (CNSs) have been recognized as advanced practice nurses (CNA, 2008) and as a result, these roles share a number of similarities. Both, for example, require education at the graduate level and share the core role competencies associated with advanced nursing practice: direct patient care, research, leadership, consultation, and collaboration (CNA, 2008). Both, under the umbrella of advanced nursing practice, are involved in "analyzing and synthesizing knowledge; understanding, interpreting and applying nursing theory and research; and developing and advancing nursing knowledge and the profession as a whole" (p. 10). However, the extent of NP and CNS involvement in the activities associated with each of the competencies has varied depending on the expectations of the administrators and physicians in the organization (Donald et al., 2010; Kilpatrick et al., 2010).

Economic discourse has concerned issues of costs of care within the context of striving for optimal outcomes, with its purpose of building a case for the use of NPs as alternative health care providers. NPs have repeatedly been promoted as an inexpensive, albeit excellent, alternative to physicians. Multiple studies in a variety of settings and patient populations have confirmed that NPs provide cost savings to the health care system (Hoffman et al., 2005; Meyer and Miers, 2005; Williams and Sidani, 2001). For example, studies have compared NPs' and physicians' care provision in terms of volume of patients seen per day, average length of hospital stay, rate of readmission, mortality and morbidity, number of drugs prescribed, diagnostic tests ordered, consultations and referrals made, correct diagnoses, days on oxygen and/or ventilator, and monthly cost of care per patient.

It becomes clear that the prime focus of discourse within these domains has been the NPs' direct clinical practice activities. Because of their link to procedural activities, their role has been strongly associated with the highly valued medical model of cure, and is easy to visualize, articulate, cost-analyze, and cost-compare. The degree of responsibility in the advanced nursing practice areas of research, education, program and policy development, quality assurance, and professional activity involvement is known to vary widely and is often a small component of the job because of direct patient-care responsibilities (D'Amour et al., 2007; Roschkov et al., 2004).

There is little critical discourse that focuses on the ontological nature of the NP role. A few nurse researchers have attempted to broaden the discussion with their studies of NPs working in the primary health care sector. Their findings reveal that NPs engage in responsible risk-taking, the skilled healing practice of personal persuasion, engagement in the mutuality of decision-making, and proficiency in the art of listening and attending (Brykczynski, 1985; Brykczynski and Lewis, 1997; Lewis and Brykczynski,

1994). These caring relationships are personal, egalitarian, and collaborative (Beal and Quinn, 2002; Brown and Draye, 2003). Such insights are just beginning to transform the understanding and study of the NP movement. The power of this emerging discourse lies in its ability to uncover some of the qualitative distinctions and commonalities in the practices of NPs and physicians, and to elucidate and give voice to NPs' unique contribution to health care. I am not suggesting that in order to strengthen this discourse we need to move away from the instrumental or economic discourses. In fact, that would be as harmful as the present situation. However, it is readily apparent that our way of knowing the NP is incomplete. Bowker, Timmermans, and Star (1995, p. 363) wrote, "A light shining in the dark illuminates certain areas of nursing work, but may cast shadows elsewhere."

As I undertook this research journey, I understood that the picture is a complex one, but that it was time to make the invisible visible. I believed that it was a matter of "getting in on the conversation" (Jardine, 1998, p. 29) in a new way, for only in this way can the conversation be kept alive, even though it may be full of conflict and ambiguity. Therefore, the pressing question that guided my work was, "What is the experience of being an acute-care NP?" I wanted to bring into fuller view the NPs' lived experience from their perspective, and to seek a deeper understanding of the nature of their nursing practice.

Connecting Voices

In order to enrich understanding of the experience of being an acute-care NP, I engaged in a qualitative method based on hermeneutic phenomenological inquiry grounded in the philosophical writings of Martin Heidegger (1962) and Hans-Georg Gadamer (1989). Although there is no actual method (i.e., technique or procedural requirements) to this type of research, Max van Manen (1997) and Patricia Benner (1994) offered methodological structures that provide a meaningful guide to the process of this methodology; therefore, my work was both descriptive and interpretive in nature.

I searched for NPs who had been working in their role for at least two years and were employed more than 20 hours per week in their NP position so that they had had time to accumulate experiences as an acute-care NP, to begin to make sense out of them, and to embody the experience of being an NP within their practices. Participants were drawn from four adult and paediatric teaching hospitals in three provinces in the central and western regions of Canada that had been employing, for more than two years, NPs who had graduated from university-based nursing programs designed to educate nurses working in NP roles in hospital environments. Once ethics approval for the study was obtained from each participating hospital's research ethics boards, I accessed the lists of NP names by various means: the professional nursing association, the institution's human resources departments, and/or nursing administrators. I then distributed letters explaining the study via intra-hospital mail, as per each institution's directives.

Twenty-six NPs volunteered to each participate in one face-to-face, audiotaped, in-depth interview, which was carried out in a quiet setting of the participant's choice, such as the participant's home or a room within the workplace away from the patient-care area. Interviews ranged in length from two to three and a half hours. I generally began each interview with the prompt, "Share with me a day in your life as an NP," and proceeded gradually, at the participant's own pace and own direction, to conversations concerning what drew him or her to the role, his or her education and learning, seminal influences that shaped him or her in the role, key relationships, accounts of what he or she found satisfying and dissatisfying about work in the course of a day, real-life clinical decision-making, and visions of his or her future.

Of the 26 women and men who volunteered to participate in the study, all but one had graduated from a designated acute-care nurse practitioner program; the one exception had been trained as a primary-care nurse practitioner. Six had initially been prepared at the graduate level to be CNSs and had worked in this role prior to further advancing their education as NPs. They presented with a diversity of ages, nursing specialties and subspecialties, educational backgrounds, years of experience, and types of previous nursing experience. They came from neonatal, pediatric, and adult critical-care units. They worked in a variety of subspecialty services, including neurology, neurosurgery, oncology, cardiology, cardiovascular surgery, nephrology/dialysis, orthopedics, family medicine, gerontology, and subspecialty services within infection control. They are, therefore, characteristic of the NP workforce in Canada in the acute-care sector (Bryant-Lukosius et al., 2007; CIHI, 2010; Hurlock-Chorostecki, van Soreren, and Goodwin, 2008).

All but two of the NPs worked full time. Six had 10 or more years of experience in the role; 10 had between five and nine years of experience; and 10 had less than five years of experience. Only one had just the required two years necessary to be involved in the study. Total years of experience in nursing ranged from 14 to 35. However, having the most years of nursing experience did not necessarily mean that a participant was the most experienced. In fact, six participants with more than 20 years of total nursing experience had less than five years in the NP role, while three of the participants had spent more than 15 of their 20-plus years of total nursing experience in this role.

Introducing the Nurse Practitioners

An understanding of the lived experience of acute-care NPs begins here with three stories. They are an amalgam of the many stories shared by the participants in this study; none relate to one particular NP. For example, consider "Paula," who earned a bachelor's degree in science, majoring in anatomy and physiology with the intention of going to work in a research laboratory. The field of health care had always been in the back of her mind, so she continued in school and trained to be a respiratory therapist. It happened that in her first job she spent a great deal of time attending to patients in a critical-care environment, in which she frequently observed that the nurses appeared to take every opportunity to involve their patients or families in the decision-making process. She was impressed that they always seemed to be concerned about what was best for each particular patient and family, even when it meant being in conflict with other members of the team. Paula reconsidered what it meant to provide health care and realized that what she envisioned for her career was more than being involved with the technical aspects of patient care. She acknowledged that she was drawn to the philosophy of nursing, the idea of treating the person as a whole, in mind-body-spirit, and soon thereafter found herself pursuing a career as a nurse. She worked in a variety of settings and nursing positions, most recently pioneering the new NP role in oncology. Paula loved the NP career path that she had chosen. When asked if she had ever regretted this choice, she quickly responded that she "wouldn't trade in her job for all the tea in China."

Unlike Paula, "Susan" was interested in nursing from an early age. As a child, she loved to play first aid, applying bandages and trying to "make the hurt go away." She attended nursing school right out of high school and, having developed a passion for the care of babies, she secured a job in a neonatal intensive-care unit immediately upon graduation. Over the years, she had held a variety of neonatal nursing positions in transport, management, and education. She felt that her nursing career was one that continually offered learning, growth, and other endless options. Susan is a neonatal NP — a role that she, too, felt she had pioneered.

Then there is "Stephen." His mother was a public-health nurse in Ethiopia, and at a young age Stephen often accompanied her on home visits or to community clinics, acting as her translator. He witnessed up close how his mother cared for and developed relationships with patients, and how she had a high degree of autonomy and responsibility. For a time, Stephen considered becoming a physician, but after various volunteer experiences in acute-care settings and in-depth conversations with various health care professionals, he realized that what he envisioned for his career was not related to providing diagnoses and treatments. He wanted to empower patients through health education, advocacy, health promotion, and counselling — all aspects of a role that he had seen his mother perform. He received a bachelor of nursing degree and then worked as a nurse in Northern Canada. Stephen is now a nurse practitioner in a gerontology subspecialty, a role that he pioneered.

Most of us in the nursing profession traverse paths that have already been well trodden by numerous others before us. We are seldom faced with charting new courses in foreign waters, discovering new worlds, or creating new roles. However, the NPs in this study considered themselves pioneers of this role in acute-care practices. Being pioneers has meant that they leave their safe harbours without navigational charts and with no straight course to follow:

> There are no handbooks on lighthouses and perils and signals for navigating on land. No prescribed routes, no updated charts, no outlines of shoals measured in feet or

fathoms, no markers at such and such a cape, no red, green, or yellow buoys, no conventions for boarding, no clear horizons for calculating latitude. (Pérez-Reverte, 2001, p. 19)

Of all the bewildering things about pioneering a new role, the absence of landmarks — what Etienne Wenger (1998) has termed *reifications* — is one of the most challenging, frustrating, and sometimes disheartening. Just as the pioneers settling the wilderness experienced the absence of landmarks, these NP pioneers have faced a new world that lacks a community of practice. This new role within the traditional world of acute health care has not yet been captured and tamed in the form of social structures that have been historically tried and tested and then gradually sanctioned and reified as true. Canadian NPs in acute-care practices, as a group, are just beginning to develop their own routines, rituals, artifacts, symbols, conventions, stories, and histories that bind them together across time and space in such a way that there is a common sense of belonging and identity.

Wenger (1998, p. 5) pointed out that we learn from our social communities at work about the practices — the shared historical and social resources, frameworks, and perspectives — of a given role, through a collective language. This way of talking enables us "to sustain mutual engagement in action." In fact, we even take for granted the way we learn and know about which enterprises within our work are deemed worthy of pursuit, of how and when our participation in those activities is recognized as competent and trustworthy by the community. That is, we learn to know when we have met the criteria that qualify us to belong. Ultimately, we take for granted that how we have changed, learned, and come to know who we are — even within our own personally created work histories — has occurred within the context of our communities of practice. Nurses who pioneer the NP role leave behind such well-established communities in order to build new ones. Typically, the NPs in my study noted that they faced this endeavour alone in their respective areas of work — an additional challenge to be overcome in their quest for a viable identity and a sense of belonging.

This does not mean that NPs develop or preserve a sense of themselves in isolation from other communities of practice with which they work. We all belong to and work alongside several such communities at any given time, and we may even share some goals and actions with a number of them. In order to fulfill the requirements of their employers and patients — no matter how disparate and vague — NPs must create a practice in order to do what needs to be done with the set of people and the communities they work with on a day-to-day basis. As Wenger (1998, p. 6) pointed out, "In spite of curriculum, discipline, and exhortation, the learning that is most personally transformative turns out to be the learning that involves membership in these communities of practice." The experiences of pioneering NPs in dealing with the various agendas of multiple communities of practice, as well as those of their patients, shape their journey. Both the eye-opening character of the novelty or foreignness of being NPs and the remembrance of the taken-for-granted familiarity of the elements of the established nursing community of practice caused many of the struggles, tensions, and battles that these NPs faced in their transformational journey.

Nurse Practitioners' Transformational Journey

One of the most famous journeys in literature is to be found in Herman Melville's *Moby Dick*. In this novel about the adventures of a wandering sailor, Melville spoke to the journey as the possibility of self and Others being realized in a much fuller sense;

the journey is about the ability to change and adapt in a more meaningful way. Melville suggested that some people are "landsmen" who only "water-gaze," leaning against the rails of piers, trying to catch a glimpse of life beyond land, beyond safe harbours, caught up in the desire to begin a new journey. But in the end, they choose to stay with what is comfortable and safe. Others, however, have deep desires and needs for something more than what their personal or work lives have to offer. Consequently, these people orient themselves toward change, yearning for something more. These people long to set sail, to embark on an adventure and experience the untried, for staying moored to the familiar and comfortable is limiting to them. Yet setting sail means leaving what is known, feeling increasingly burdened with uncertainty, facing fears and confronting challenges, and then forging a new self-identity as they let go of old ways of being and belonging. But we are also warned that upon our return to the harbour, we are faced with the challenge of explaining what we have seen and experienced in a new way to those who want to see only what they have known from the pier.

Becoming an NP involves a journey from one mode of being as a nurse to another: from being disallowed to engage in a set of activities authorized only to physicians to being legally engaged in these activities. At first glance, this appears fairly simple. However, attention to the journey itself reveals elements of a transformative process embedded in a dialectical experience. Indeed, the NPs' journey is directed both outward, into the world, and inward, into the self. The journey outward is a series of triumphs and conflicts encountered along the way. The journey inward is a series of struggles within oneself, culminating in a union with the forces against which one struggles. For example, on the one hand, NPs are not satisfied with the traditional model within which they are required to deliver nursing care in the acute-care setting. They do not want to embody Homer's Penelope, waiting patiently, endlessly weaving and undoing the same pattern. They need to embark on their own journey in order to find a way to fully embrace their potential and value themselves as nurses. On the other hand, there is the constant danger of seeing the activities of diagnosing and prescribing as the major identifying characteristics of being an NP — and, indeed, the primary reason for the role's existence. They do not want to be seen as physician substitutes, simply an advanced model of handmaidens in the physician-dominated health care profession. Consequently, theirs is a very important journey toward being a fully integrated, balanced, and whole person within a new nursing role in the acute-care system.

The NPs' journey is not linear or unidirectional. A linear view does not account for the intertwining, dynamic, and iterative nature of the learning, growing, doing, struggling, and accommodating within relationships to be found in this journey. Nor does such a view accommodate the depth of change that this journey entails. New experiences reach back to earlier experiences, which are now understood in a different way. Similarly, earlier experiences reach forward to envelop present experiences with transformed significance. Some transformations are dramatic, but most are of an insidious and cumulative nature resulting from day-to-day experiences. For some, the transformative journey takes longer or is more intense than for others. Some NPs begin to sense their dependence and vulnerability in new ways and to doubt their abilities, and therefore feel ambivalent about the magnitude of change in their lives.

The NP's journey is not a definitive or fixed experience. For some NPs it may be a never-ending process, changing and developing with various events that they experience. Phases or periods in the journey often overlap. But ultimately, the transformative journey opens up previously unimagined new selves, new areas of responsibility, fatigue, anxiety, ambivalence, satisfaction, and joy. Just as Ishmael, the sailor in Melville's *Moby Dick*, becomes who he is as a result of wounding and healing processes, NPs learn to let go of their old ways of being and belonging, and as a result their journey becomes existential. Once this transformation occurs, their self-conceptions become harmonized with their duties, and they fulfill the Nietzschean charge to "become who you are." In a Hegelian view, this journey requires a circular perspective. It has no beginning and no end: everything finds its place and is understood as an integral aspect of a whole.

In this book, the journey is the unifying theme that links the chapters in the participants' stories of their ways of being and becoming NPs working in acute-care practices, and of the long transformational process that they must make if they are to claim the power of their own minds, voices, and practices. In describing their lived experience, these NPs commonly used metaphors involving water: "paddling as fast as I can," "keeping my head above water," "treading water," "being thrown a lifeline," "murky water," "calm waters," "feeling adrift," and so on. Wherever possible, I have attempted to maintain this metaphor in keeping with their voices, just as I have used their words to title the various themes and meaning units of the journey. This book is as much about the NPs' pain, frustration, and fear as it is about their finding professional satisfaction. At the time of the interviews, a few NPs were in the midst of considering professional change, and they shared with me both recent and distant transitional experiences that had shaped the way they perceived themselves and the world around them. Not all of the stories were happy ones. This book is also about "the roar which lies on the other side of silence" (Eliot, 2002, p. 185) — the opportunity to have the acute-care NP voices heard in a new way, to help to make the discourse about who they are and what they do more complete.

In the first chapter, the journey begins with nurses' desire to search for something more in who they can be as nurses and what they can offer to others — the search for being more connected, more in control, more visible, more challenged, and being able to make more of a difference in their nursing practice. This beginning requires either the seizing or creating of an opportunity, with the NP role perceived as possibly offering "the perfect fit." Chapter 2 tells the story of the NPs' turbulent journey through the uncertain waters of engaging in medical responsibilities previously denied them in other nursing roles, a time of being adrift, experienced as being disconnected, uncertain, and lost, but also of staying afloat. In chapter 3, the story shifts to the emergence of NPs' feelings of inner security that emerge from being competent, confident, and comfortable in their performance of the various elements of their clinical practice, which opens the way for being committed, connected, and content. During this part of their journey, NPs fully sense their direct clinical practice role. Chapter 4 reveals that the journey is not yet over. NPs discuss new tensions that arise from the shift in internally or externally driven performance expectations in other dimensions of their role as advanced practice nurses; a time during which they experience being pulled to be "more." In chapter 5, a further transformational process is revealed: that of being more, experienced as being an advanced practitioner. At this point in their journey some NPs experience the unification of the direct practice, research, leadership, consultation, and collaboration competencies of the advanced nursing practice role.

Despite being burdened by a struggle enmeshed with politics and history, NPs eventually navigate their own course as they journey toward self-knowledge, personal transformation, and authentic living as a nurse. Consequently, they experience an odyssey of learning — learning to find a new place where they feel they belong, learning to engage in and contribute to their communities of practice in a new way, and learning to inhabit a new identity — all of which are part of the quest for more, for finding the perfect fit.

Steps slowed
Head bent low
But still along the way

Hopelessness pervaded
Doubts persuaded
But still along the way

Time and again
Fear shouted "You're no man"
But still along the way

Sweat and tears
Poured through years
But still along the way

Stumbling, crawling
Crying out, calling
But still along the way

Searching blindly
For destination and finally
Finding it one glorious day

— **Jana Justice-Olivieri**, "The Journey"

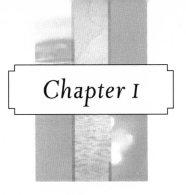

Chapter I

Being Called To Be More

A journey of a thousand miles must begin with a single step.
— Lao Tzu

Why do nurses decide to become NPs? What initiates or precipitates their journey? What are they looking for? What might they be running away from or toward? What more do they want? How do they know when to start out?

Certainly, the call to be an NP is not always clearly heard or understood at first, and for many the destination is also unclear. Some nurses take the leap without a moment's hesitation, while others lag behind, watching the experience of others and then following their lead. For some, the desire to be an NP is driven by a vague pull toward something more. Not quite satisfied with who they are as nurses or what they are currently doing, they are willing to test new waters and set sail for destinations unknown, unsure of what they are looking for but hoping that it will be revealed along the way. Nevertheless, knowing what they value and what they no longer want becomes their North Star. For others, setting out on the journey begins with a dream: they are motivated to pioneer the NP role and continue to be fortified during the journey by reflecting on what it could mean to patients or nursing. Their reflections bring them to a new consciousness of nursing; they are almost able to feel a new relationship with it.

"Joan" worked as a CNS in a program whose patient population had outgrown the number of staff members that could effectively provide the complex clinical service needed. It came to her attention that the provincial government was looking to fund programs that would deliver health care in innovative ways. Joan used this external call as the opportunity to submit a proposal for a five-person interdisciplinary team — composed of a physician, an NP, a social worker, a pharmacist, and a clinic nurse — that would deliver one-stop care to the patients in the program. She lobbied across the institution for the NP position, with herself in the role, seeking support from the service's clinical team members including the medical and administrative directors. In her own words, what Joan really wanted to do "was to be able to marry the kind of things that are called physician practice, things that the physicians are felt to be responsible for, and bring them into [her] nursing practice" and "really focus in on a certain group of individuals who [she] felt were falling through the cracks in our health care system." The new program received funding, and the group, with Joan as NP, provided holistic care for the province's entire specific patient population (approximately 900 people) from 2001 on.

For nurses like Joan, the dream of being an NP is fairly detailed: they are weaving careers from their dreams, setting out to find or create a nursing role that is the perfect fit. As weavers of their roles, some nurses first create a mental picture of their destiny as NPs — a vision of who they want to be and what they want to accomplish. They select the patterns, colours, and textures of their lives in this role. It is up to them to judge how pleased they are and to decide what changes are needed in order to create their desired role. Being a pioneer makes this creation possible, and the vision becomes the sextant used to navigate their journey.

This is not to say that the nurses' dreams or desires include a navigational chart, or even what the exact destination will look like. Yet whether they are visionaries or seekers, as they struggle to find a place within their clinical program, organization, and profession as NPs, they find that their desire for more is what they need to help them deal with the tensions and turbulence they experience throughout their journey. The constant refocusing and reflecting on what first called them to the NP role in the first place helps them to visualize the difference that they wish to make, the people whom they want to help, and the goals that they hope to achieve. Ultimately, their desire for more helps them determine when they have reached their personal destination of being an NP.

In seizing the opportunity to become an NP, nurses perceive possibilities for who they can be as nurses and what they can bring to their nursing practice that they may not have seen in any other nursing role. They have found only a partial fit with who they want to be as nurses but are hopeful that the NP role will offer a perfect fit. Being in direct clinical practice is an integral part of that fit. For at the heart of being an NP is, as one NP noted, "the opportunity to work with patients, hands on, all the time." For nurses already in patient-care roles (e.g., bedside or transport nurses), the NP role offers the possibility of being more in clinical practice without requiring that they leave the profession. For those who have been away from hands-on care, becoming an NP offers the possibility of returning to that which they love and miss but combining it with the opportunity to include more of that which they have found in other nursing roles (e.g., administrative leadership or education).

The desire for more is inherent in the reasons for initiating the journey to become an NP. "Kerry," a neonatal NP, had worked in a variety of settings over the course of her twenty-five-year nursing career — obstetrics, pediatrics, public health — intertwined with various stretches back at school. Yet, she had always come back to the neonatal area. She had pioneered a neonatal transport program and she loved the autonomy that it provided. The attraction was the critical thinking needed on transport, the ability to put the pieces of the puzzle together. Kerry loved making a diagnosis, finding the solution, and working collaboratively with her medical colleagues. But she realized that she was still not fully satisfied; she wanted more. The transport role had whet her appetite for the possibilities of what more she could be and do as a nurse, what more she was capable of, and what more she could offer to the patients. She discovered possibilities within herself for being as a nurse that she liked and desired, and she chose to bring them into the light. When the prospect arose for her to pioneer the NP role, she felt that it provided the opportunity for her to learn more, maximize her potential, and contribute and make a broader difference to patients, their families, and nurses at the bedside. At the same time, it would complement who she already was as a nurse.

There are five dominant forces for being called to be more: being more connected, being more in control, being more visible, being more challenged, and being able to make more of a difference. Rarely is only one of these forces involved in the process.

Being More Connected

Being connected, physically and emotionally, to patients and families is a strong force for becoming an NP. "Laura" had worked in a cardiology clinic where she enjoyed being recognized as an arrhythmia expert. She also cherished the freedom bestowed upon her by the physicians to detect and diagnose pacemaker dysrhythmias and to reprogram them as necessary to fix the problem. However, she felt that she had become very technical in her nursing role. Laura felt a loss of nursing and so returned to an inpatient bedside nursing role in which she could feel more connected to the patients and their families. Yet in this role she felt the loss of self-sufficiency and recognition that she had formerly experienced. Consequently she was searching for something more when an NP program at the local university opened its doors. Laura knew immediately that it was what she wanted to do. Others similarly described being in clinical management or clinical educator positions as being too far away from patients. As one NP noted, the role opened the possibility of "being able to combine teaching with team leadership and a bit of research, while allowing me to stay close to the patient. This is a good fit for me. It gives me all of the things that I think are important about nursing."

Establishing meaningful connections with patients and their families and being involved in a personal way is at the heart of caring and commitment in nursing. Bishop and Scudder (1990) found that even if individuals are not initially attracted to nursing for this reason, the sense of connectedness becomes embedded in their personal sense of nursing if they choose to remain in the profession. "Abby" recalled how restless she had become in her work as a clinical educator, in large part because she was afraid she had begun to move too far away from the bedside. The driving force behind her decision to pioneer the NP role had been to be more personally connected with patients and families, while still being able to connect with and make a difference to her immediate nursing colleagues in the education component of the role. In addition, she could make larger systemic changes within nursing, something that she had experienced as an infection-control nurse. As Abby continued in her reflections, she revealed the circular nature of her nursing journey: "It's fascinating to go back and look at where your career path has taken you and the steps that you took that you weren't sure where they were going to lead, but in fact, in hindsight, do lead up to you integrating those skills."

Having worked as a candy striper during her adolescence, Abby had been drawn to the sciences. But even at that time, she knew she would not enjoy the episodic nature of their patient-care service: "I didn't want to be in a position of just popping in and popping out. I wanted to actually understand and develop relationships with people over a longer period of time." Instead, nursing provided her with the opportunity to be with patients and families over a longer duration and to be immersed in learning the sciences. However, the traditional bedside nursing role had ultimately not been challenging or autonomous enough for her — hence the sojourns in other nursing roles that took her away from hands-on clinical practice, the only alternatives at the time. The creation of the NP role finally offered Abby the possibility of being intellectually challenged in the multiple dimensions of nursing, while at the same time being more intimately connected with patients and families over long periods.

Being More in Control

Majestic eagle
In gilded cage, her wings clipped
Her spirit sundered.

— Mika Yoshimoto (2008, p. 6)

Some nurses are strongly attracted by the possibility of finally having both increased responsibilities and the autonomy to act in their clinical practice. In other words, they seek to have control over their practices, which they feel has been missing from or has eluded them in their role as bedside nurses. Indeed, the frustrations with practice limitations and the inability to experience their own potential in the traditional bedside nursing role has led many nurses to consider either applying to medical school or leaving the health care field altogether. However, the NP role offers them the opportunity to remain rooted in the nursing profession, in direct clinical practice, in a position that holds the promise that they can have more independence and more control over the decisions about patient care, including the treatment plan and the way in which the care can be delivered. Greater knowledge and skill, combined with the authority to use all of their abilities more holistically, potentially enables nurses to make a greater difference, a finding equally expressed by a group of American primary-care NP pioneers in the mid-1960s and throughout the 1970s (Brown and Draye, 2003). One NP explained her attraction to the role:

> At the time I was in a staff role and I wanted to do something
> different. . . . The focus wasn't on delivering the best patient care,
> it was on who has the appropriate title to do X amount of care. Just
> one example: a patient has a headache. As a nurse you've certainly
> got the knowledge and expertise to know they need Tylenol but
> you can't give them Tylenol until you call the physician to get
> an order for plain Tylenol. I found that kind of thing incredibly
> frustrating because it wasn't a matter of the nurse not having the
> knowledge and expertise; it was the role limitations, the barriers
> to optimal practice. So the patient's suffering while you're jumping
> through these hoops to get something that the nurse should be
> able to deliver. . . . So I thought to myself, I either jump ship or

go into medicine, which didn't really appeal to me because I love nursing. . . . And I finally decided that . . . I was going to stick it out but I would do my masters preparation, which would give me the background to have more options. And at that time the NP role had been piloted at [hospital] . . . they were trying new territory . . . and I decided that it might just fit for me.

Suzanne Gordon's journalistic work, Nursing Against the Odds (2005), passionately describes the health care systems that severely restrict what nurses can do without a doctor's order, which both creates problems and reinforces status and power hierarchies between nurses and physicians, a deadly catch-22 situation. She described this situation from the physician's perspective:

Every night, a thousand times a night, all over the country, nurses are calling doctors reporting that a patient has a fever and asking doctors what they should do about it, or asking the doctor whether they should give the patient Tylenol. And every night, doctors are berating nurses for calling them up and bothering them, because they are reporting a fever, and the doctors are thinking to themselves, "Why are you so stupid that you are asking me whether you should give Tylenol?" (p. 48)

Akin to wanting more control is the desire for more flexibility. Wanting to be more involved in all aspects of the patient's care ("the social, the emotional, helping patients cope with the stressors, the medical care"), liking the flexibility in meeting the patients' needs, and appreciating the additional responsibility and accountability results in nurses being attracted to a role in which they believe they will be able to direct care in collaboration with physicians. Moreover, they are drawn to the possibility of being able to spend time with patients and their families.

Being More Visible

It was about diagnosing and coming up with the solution and being able to really work collaboratively and build those partnerships with our medical colleagues. . . . And I felt as a nurse that one of the opportunities to present itself would be to become a neonatal nurse practitioner. . . . Well I guess, it's like that power, not power, but the sense of fulfilment that you have at the bedside when you work together . . . being part of the team in terms of how could I, as a nurse practitioner, be more part of . . . working collaboratively with making that plan . . . but working with the nurse, working with the whole team in how we can make a difference, but really being part of that discussion.

Becoming an NP is also about the call to be more visible: the search for a more collaborative practice, of being able to contribute more to the team and to experience the feeling of being truly valued, all inherently speak to this. Nurses who become NPs want to have their voices heard and to be recognized and acknowledged for their own agency. They are frustrated with being viewed as "just a nurse" (an implication that nurses are engaged in insignificant work) or "just temporarily borrowing the doctor's agency" (Gordon, 2005, p. 50). NPs view their role as an opportunity to be affirmed and recognized for what they know and do, rather than having their actions attributed to the physician. For instance, "Sally," in her role of transport nurse, was tired of the evasive and roundabout language that demonstrates deference to physicians. She no longer wanted to play the doctor–nurse game of arriving at the identification of the problem or plan of care without venturing on the medical territory of diagnosis, treatment, or prescribing:

So you have an air leak happening and the baby's telling you what symptoms he's having; you're looking at an X-ray that's telling you, this baby has a pneumothorax. And the parents are asking me,

"Well why are you putting that needle in the chest?" And so, you're going, "Well he has symptoms that are suggestive of a hole in his lung, an air leak." No. He's got a pneumothorax. It's a diagnosis. It just boggles my mind to try and get the wordsmithing around just to stay within the scope of nursing.

Gordon (2005) observed that even in settings in which nurses can change ventilator settings, wean patients off inotropic agents, insert catheters, and initiate intravenous fluid therapy, after which they get the physician (resident) to write an order, the treatment interventions are presented on rounds in such a way that the nurse seems to have acted on the physician's behalf. As these participants confirmed, it is common to hear staff physicians inform new residents that nurses know their preferences. All of this reinforces what physicians admit that they have been taught through informal or formal lessons and socialization: "The nurse is stupid, because she uses dumb language, makes dumb suggestions, and doesn't know anywhere near what the physician knows" (Gordon, 2005, p. 49). Nurses "have no real agency of their own" (p. 50).

The term *doctor–nurse games* was coined by Leonard Stein (1967) to refer to the implicit or explicit relationships of power between physicians and nurses and the social game played by both parties to maintain that balance. Such "games" conceal nurses' mastery of their knowledge and skills and their importance to patients. Nurses remain barely visible to physicians, except as objects of derision and disrespect. One participant bemoaned that nurses are visible to society only as individuals who carry a bedpan for a living. According to Gordon (2005, p. 148), nurses continue to be viewed as individuals "who operate on a field that has already been prepared for them by the doctor."

In Hegel's (1971) parable of the master and the slave, presented in *Phenomenology of Mind*, two individuals approach each other from opposite directions along a path. As they approach each other, they desire recognition — for they do not really know who they are until they see themselves in another's eyes, until they are recognized by an Other. They desire the recognition of one person by another as equal human beings. Yet each fears that the Other will deny him this recognition, will force him to submit to his will by moving off the path. So, they fight until one submits. In this story, Hegel informs us that our very sense of who we are — our identity — is constructed in relation to the Other and has no autonomous meaning. For example, I cannot be a master, act as and think of myself as a master, unless the slave acts toward me as slave to master and treats me as a master. And vice versa for the slave. For Hegel, consciousness (one's sense of self; one's identity) is always limited by its embeddedness in history, and thus neither the master nor the slave is able to think outside the modes of consciousness that are available in the culture at a particular point in time. It could be argued, then, that if nurses are never able to rise outside the history and positionality of nursing as it is currently constituted in our culture, they will remain invested in their historical role as the physicians' handmaiden, a position perceived as unequal and lacking in recognition and freedom. Hegel further proposes that the process of recognition is "a battle" (p. 171), a "life and death struggle" (p. 172). Charles Taylor (1994, p. 50), a Canadian philosopher, explicitly draws on Hegel to argue that "the struggle for recognition can find only one satisfactory solution, and that is a regime of reciprocal recognition among equals." Yet Hegel (1971) proposes that for the slave,

> who has not the courage to risk his life to win freedom, that man deserves to be a slave; on the other hand, if a nation does not merely imagine that it wants to be free but actually has the energy to will its freedom, then no human power can hold it back in the servitude of a merely passive obedience to authority. (p. 175)

Viewing freedom from this Hegelian perspective, is it possible that nurses who wish to be NPs have perceived the physician-nurse relationship as an asymmetrical one such as that of master and slave, and that, by remaining in this traditional relationship, they will be unable to experience a full flourishing nursing life? Is it possible that nurses who wish to be NPs recognize this pioneering journey as an opportunity to be active agents of culture and history, shaping what nursing can be, and therefore act in ways that lead to the recognition that has previously been denied nurses and nursing?

Being More Challenged

A lot of the excitement is in making the diagnosis, in the seeking of information, putting the clues together. . . . And part of it is the inquisitiveness or the intuition that takes you to the next step — Have you thought of? Did you? Would this have made a difference? Why are we doing things the way we're doing them? . . . I was ready for another challenge, another learning opportunity.

Thomas Henry Huxley wrote, "The rung of a ladder was never meant to rest upon, but only to hold a man's foot long enough to enable him to put the other somewhat higher" (Bartlett and Kaplan, 1992). Some nurses, once they possess a sense of ease with the nursing terrain they have already explored, are challenged to extend the horizons of their actions and risk their stable identity for a different identification with their world. They seek to feel more challenged in their practice, more stimulated in their work, and more motivated that they can continually grow and learn as nurses. Although this can be accomplished by transferring to another type of specialty nursing, advancing one's education, or moving into an administrative, education, or research role, none of these options was perceived as the perfect fit for those nurses seeking a multiplicity of "mores" while engaging in direct patient care.

A desire for personal growth, woven into a need to be challenged and to feed one's inquisitive nature, to expand one's wings, is another common thread among NPs. Indeed, many participants expressed a sense of good fortune and gratitude at having had mentors along the way who saw their potential, encouraged them, and provided opportunities to push themselves. The mentors spoke to the individuals' desire to maximize their potential, although many were uncertain of their capabilities when they initiated their journey. As one NP noted, the NP role is perceived as initiating the opportunity to be able to continually move, which is the perfect fit for someone who loves to study and wants to constantly strive for more knowledge and skills that can be used at the bedside, close to the patients and their families. The role provides more academic and clinical educational opportunities, thus offering the potential for NPs to challenge their intellectual abilities, and revealing the multiple possibilities for being a nurse in clinical practice.

Some NPs are strongly attracted to the scientific focus of medicine. Some expressed this as a desire to study more anatomy and physiology in particular, or the study of math, biology, chemistry, and physics, although they were reticent to frankly admit to something that is now deemed to be politically incorrect in nursing — an outcome, intended or not, of the discourse of nursing scholars such as Gail Mitchell and Marc Santopinto (1998), Martha Rogers (1972), and Margaret Sandelowski (2000). The NPs had chosen less depth of knowledge in the hard-core sciences in order to achieve the broader perspective of human life and the human condition that nursing offered. A desire to learn more technical skills, to be mentally stimulated by the complex problem-solving inherent in making a diagnosis, and to feel that they are doing something that's making a difference to someone's care in terms of their biological status, was, as several NPs noted, a real incentive for them. Yet, the acknowledgment of being drawn to this level of knowledge and skill is always embedded in the recognition that this is not nearly enough for them in their practice. They envision that becoming an NP will give them that little extra they want, in terms of more knowledge and skill, embedded within a connected relationship to their patients and families. "It really is an ideal role," summarized one NP, "that offers the opportunity to attain more depth in the medical sciences, which, when combined with nursing knowledge, better enables nurses to meet the patients' needs in a more timely and holistic manner."

Some nurses are enticed by the opportunity to integrate many different aspects of practice, to feel, in some NPs' words, "more well-rounded." This appears to be particularly true for NPs who have held a diversity of nursing roles throughout their careers. One NP explained why she had been drawn to the role:

> Being able to bring all of the experiences that I've had throughout my career, being able to work with a variety of people, being able to make a difference at the bedside, but also being able to do some of those other more advanced practice roles, being able to go to conferences, present, publish, do research, mentor colleagues, being able to interact with different people, different organizations — I think all of those things were really critical for me.

Finally, for some nurses there is the call toward leaving that which is familiar in order to explore uncharted territory; the challenge of being a pioneer is, in and of itself, an exciting opportunity to test one's abilities, creativity, and initiative. Itching to develop and use their full expertise and potential, these nurses exemplify what it means to risk what is known in order to open up to new possibilities for the purpose of securing a greater hold on their world within nursing. One NP explained, "I really felt it was important to move along and see myself as taking on a challenge that not many people have taken. So I felt I was one of the first people that saw the nurse practitioner [role] as a way to expand my wings and went for it and got in and it was just really exciting to be moving in a new direction."

Traditionally, nurses have been socialized to be nice, to be compliant. Perhaps this socialization can be viewed as "shrink to fit": shrinking oneself to fit what others expect. As Brown and Draye (2003) found — a finding confirmed in these participants' stories — the NPs' struggle is for autonomy not for its own sake but as a means to transcend the limitations in the traditional bedside nursing role. They are in search of a new fit that challenges their personal abilities and provides the opportunities to discover their own possibilities for being.

Being Able to Make More of a Difference

A desire to deepen, broaden, and strengthen one's knowledge, skills, and abilities regarding the medical aspects of patients' care, matched with authorized application (which is associated with being more in control), is intimately linked to a desire to provide more effective and holistic nursing care. The NP role, perceived as offering the opportunity to know the patient's clinical condition in greater depth, speaks to a practitioner's desire to better understand the patients' underlying disease processes and have a larger repertoire of tools and skills with which to help the patients and their families. NPs envision that the additional knowledge and skill will enable them to make more of a difference.

Waiting is part of the lived experience of being a nurse. Nurses wait for the physician to be of the same mind regarding the needs of the patient as brought forward by the nurse on behalf of the patient or family. They live with having to wait for physicians to respond to patient care needs: "Nothing bothers me more than to see a patient writhing in pain while the nurse is struggling to get hold of a physician who won't answer his page or having to wait until the physician gets out of the operating room, or whatever they're tied up doing, before the patient gets an analgesic." Becoming an NP includes the vision of being able to provide more timely care.

Arising from the increasing fragmentation of care in the modern health system is a vision of being able to provide consistency and continuity of care over time, rather than the snapshot, episodic, or sporadic contacts that tend to occur within the medical model of care in the hospital setting. Achieving this vision will better facilitate meeting the holistic and multiple health care needs of patients and their families:

> [W]e were talking about bringing in a care provider, a physician, who could be some doc from a doctor's office, or a replacement who'd come through the city who didn't know our babies well, maybe didn't have a whole understanding of neonatology, and definitely not the dynamics of neonatal programs and family-centred care and developmental care, just the general pathologies that we see in the neonatal population. We have nurses working at the bedside who are experts, who do have an understanding of those, working with our families day to day with certain groups of babies. And yet we were having strangers come in and look after them and write the orders. And here was an opportunity for nurses — and the literature supported that nurses could be given the education [as an NP] and be able to be that care taker . . . [who] know our babies and provide the continuity of care, the consistency of the relationship with the families.

The NP role offers the opportunity to make change for patients and families not only in relation to the patients' biological needs, but also in terms of the variety of other needs, such as quality-of-life issues, that are present as a result of physical illness. It is also seen as an opportunity to utilize creativity and initiative in new and expanded ways to bring about system-wide change that may result in better service to patients and their families.

Some nurses, particularly those who have been in CNS positions, are also drawn to the possibility of making a difference to the nurses with whom they work and the nursing profession as a whole, while retaining a focus of clinical practice at the same time. There is a strong desire to greatly help the staff nurses by connecting teaching, research, and leadership with advanced nursing care at the bedside. One NP reflected that she felt the role offered a greater chance to demonstrate to junior nurses a whole spectrum of options in the clinical setting, as it is now rare for nurses to stay in one area for 25 years. She hoped that by being a role model for her nursing colleagues, she would be able to heighten others' awareness of what nursing brings to patients and families, and thus retain nurses at the bedside and attract others into the nursing profession.

Answering the Call: Initiating the Journey

It is not always easy to hear the voice from within, let alone heed it. But once it is noticed, some form of action is required. At this point, some nurses may decline to journey further. Even when they gain a fresh insight into their discontent, they may swat it away like an annoying fly. Others disperse this uncomfortable energy by talking about it incessantly, and so they never gather and hold the energy to do anything about it. But some nurses say yes to the call. They seize or create opportunities to initiate their quest in search of more, even though it is at this point that saying yes to the journey means facing the first challenge: fear of commitment to a journey with an unknown destination. Commitment, in fact, can be quite sobering. In answering the call, they must step into the uncertain waters of the unknown and enter the sea of risk. Yet saying yes to the journey is an invocation that can connect them to all those who believe in its power, and once they are ready to commit, opportunities and circumstances seem to open in a most serendipitous unfolding.

In the history of nursing, in both Canada and the United States, many nurses have seized an opportunity to follow their dreams as a result of questions and concerns about the lack of resident coverage in the academic teaching hospitals. Pioneering NPs in acute-care practices have been privy to the debate about who can and should best fill the service gap, through discussions with their immediate supervisors, many of whom have been recognized and acknowledged as visionaries. For some nurses in this study, the desire for change and personal growth, particularly in the direct clinical practice arena, had been present for many years. However, without the creation of the NP role in this setting by nursing visionaries, they may have remained as bedside nurses, turned to management or teaching, or left nursing altogether.

And [the Nursing Department] felt that what they needed to do was to look at the clinical gaps in the hospital around the resident, but also around nursing. On the surgical floors one of the gaps they felt that there was, was accessibility to surgeons during the day because they were in the operating room, or in clinics, and [the nurses] couldn't reach them and so there were communication gaps. . . . They felt there needed to be more nurse education, there needed to be more mentoring and nurse experts in the building; so the role came about with looking at all those gaps. . . . I was in the right place at the time . . . and I was ready for a change.

It is equally important that there are visionary physicians who embrace the role. These pioneering NPs were cognizant of their "good fortune" in working with physician colleagues who were not threatened by the idea of sharing their practice knowledge with nurses in a new role, and who viewed the NP role as a possible collaboration, not a replacement for residents.

During the 1990s, hospitals all across Canada reduced the number of CNSs or phased out the role entirely. Some nurses chose to become NPs because they either heard unsettling rumours of change or were forthrightly informed that their CNS positions were to be declared redundant; they needed to change with the times. CNSs felt lucky when their nursing directors guarded their welfare by suggesting that they combine the CNS and NP roles. Some were fully supported financially to obtain the additional NP educational qualifications, while others had staff physicians who assisted them in securing clinical internship placements. They chose to seize the opportunity to pursue advanced knowledge and skills as a means to augment their effectiveness. Similarly, nurses returning to school for a graduate degree in the hope of opening up other career opportunities suddenly found acute-care, hospital-based NP programs being offered to them. Other nurses who had left the clinical area in search of new challenges as clinical educators, managers, and research assistants jumped at the opportunity to return to direct clinical practice when they were approached or supported by their nursing leaders or physician colleagues to create an NP position in their area of expertise. In one narrative, a physician not only encouraged the nurse to become an NP, but also made it a realistic venture for her. In addition to making it possible for her to return to school full time while working flex hours in her full-time position, he helped to create an environment of support among all the physicians within the service, and then mentored her during the clinical practicum.

Sometimes the opportunity comes in the form of a personal invitation to join the pioneering team. Such external recognition from a reliable and respected source prompts nurses to consider the possibility that they might be able to take on this new challenge. Without this recognition, many doubt that they would ever have considered such an undertaking, let alone believed they were capable of such an endeavour. As "Caitlyn" admitted, her first response when asked to consider applying for a temporary NP position was "to go into the corner to the other nurse clinicians and say, 'Do you think I can do this?'" Encouraged by another NP in the institution, Caitlyn found the courage to test the waters. Surprisingly, she said that she had initially left bedside nursing because of a lack of confidence in her own abilities and an overwhelming fear that she would harm her patients because of her perceived lack of appropriate knowledge and skills. Anticipating that she would have to leave nursing altogether, she had been offered clinical project work, a job that helped her to see the bigger picture and think system wide. In this position, she met others who recognized her potential and encouraged her to return to the bedside as an NP. Caitlyn had been an NP for nearly a decade at the time of my interview.

Many nurses also develop the confidence and courage to enroll in graduate school, pioneer the NP role in their institutions, and persevere when the journey becomes particularly treacherous, the obstacles overwhelming, and the number of battles lost outnumber those won, because an Athena has supported them in challenging the status quo early in their nursing careers. "Jill" recollected that as part of her consolidation experience, she had spent a month in an outpost nursing facility, where she witnessed an expanded-role nurse in action. There she had the opportunity to see and do things that she would never have seen and done in the city. This experience encouraged her to be a risk-taker and independent thinker. She also noted that at the beginning of her nursing career, she had worked for a wonderful head nurse who strove to develop a strong sense of professional nursing identity and patient-care responsibility in each staff member by instituting primary nursing care, a nursing orientation that she believed she would find once again in the NP role. This mentor had a "maybe we could" philosophy that Jill found empowering and that helped to "set her up for down the road." This "can do" message is one that some nurses hear throughout their personal and/or professional lives, providing them with the impetus necessary to seize the day when it finally presents itself and to initiate the journey.

In summary, it is often because of the encouragement of others that nurses who initiate the NP journey are willing to explore the possibility of answering the call. These leaders are perceived as wings-beneath-their-feet mentors, leaders whose message is always, "If you believe in something, do it. Don't worry about things, have integrity, but don't not do something because you think that you can't." Inspiring nurses to dream big, take risks, and to believe in themselves, to see their abilities and their potential, these leaders are the winds necessary to help them set sail. And so the journey begins.

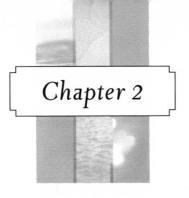

Chapter 2

Being Adrift

tangled in
sinking wreckage
of present.
anchored to
disillusionment
of dying past.
adrift on
engulfing tide
of future
with flagging sails set
in no particular direction.

— Jana Justice-Olivieri, "Adrift"

"In the port is safety, comfort, hearthstone, supper, warm blankets, friends, all that's kind to our mortalities" (Melville, 1992, p. 116). Melville begins his epic novel *Moby Dick* in the safe harbours of New Bedford, a town that exists as a place of departure and return for whaling boats. In the harbour, everyday life is intelligible and predictable. The daily routines and rituals provide a terra firma. Melville suggests that safe harbours are places where people anchor themselves in what is comfortable and secure, in a fixed sense of who they are, either as members of the dominant culture or as others given a space at the margins.

Nursing, as known by NPs prior to initiating their NP journey, is like New Bedford, a particular type of community: safe and secure in itself, with most of them absorbed in the everydayness of their lives. Work life is predictable. Yet in order to grow and develop, to realize their fuller possibilities, like Melville's protagonist Ishmael, nurses who become acute-care NPs are those who become weary of comfortable spaces and are prepared to sacrifice the safety of the harbour and venture forth. Once they commit themselves to the journey, however, they are cast adrift; as Melville metaphorically observes in the narrative of Ishmael's journey, "In the gale, the port, the land, is the ship's direst jeopardy" (p. 116).

Patient care by NPs requires sophisticated skills, advanced critical thinking abilities, political savvy, and a high level of decision-making, and thus necessitates their full focus and energies. For the most part, nurses who embark on the journey are confident and expert in the nursing roles they are leaving. When they commit to the launch, they must leave this comforting port of competence and enter a new position with different and unknown expectations. Because the NP role continues to evolve over time, and is influenced by many environmental factors both internal and external to the hospital setting, their journey is barely beginning upon completion of their formal NP training. Certainly, as students, they will have had experience making diagnostic and treatment decisions. However, as noted by Buehler (1987, p. 50), these are made as a "guest" in training sites and with full recognition that they are, after all, "only" learning. New NPs face the major tests of their clinical judgment in their first positions. Being adrift then is a time of transition.

The work of cultural anthropologists Arnold van Gennep (1960) and Victor Turner (1969, 1974, 1984) on rites of passage helps us to find meaning in NPs' experience of being adrift. In his book *The Rites of Passage*, van Gennep distinguished three stages of transition. During the initial stage, a person is separated from his status in society. This leads to the second stage, a marginal and liminal state, or state of ambiguity, which has none of the attributes of the past or future states. After an initiation, the person is finally reintegrated into the social structure in a newly achieved role-status, the third, or post-liminal, stage. Viewed from this perspective, journeying through "being adrift" is the NPs' experience of the second transitional stage; that is, literal or symbolic removal from normal patterns engenders the NPs' experience of marginality or liminality.

the place/spacetime
the situation/
leaning on the membrane between one dimension and
the next you will find it flexible as well as transparent.
moving between dimensions requires a leap of faith.

— Peter Beckett (2009), "Luminality"

Liminality, sometimes referred to as luminality, has etymological connections with words such as limit, limbo, preliminary, sublime, and subliminal (Barnhart, 1988). As the Latin root of these words limen, meaning "threshold or boundary," implies, NPs find themselves "betwixt and between" social categories and states of being. Turner referred to people in this place as "threshold people" (Turner,

1969), living in "a place that is not a place, and a time that is not a time" (Turner, 1974, p. 239), as if they were in a tunnel between the "entrance" and the "exit" (Turner, 1974, p. 231).

New NPs experience a sense of being disconnected, which may involve both a physical and mental separation. In many cases there is simply a mental separation as the NP still engages in some of the regular nursing activities. For them, the liminal state incorporates a time and space in which they are transitioning from being in a nursing role assigned traditional laws, customs, and conventions to being in a role that has new and different laws, customs, and conventions. Therese Schroeder-Sheker (1994, p. 92) described this state as a "scared condition in and out of time, where bonds between people ignore, reverse, cut across, or occur outside structural relationship." Liminal activities tend to be extreme; they appear strange, and sometimes disturbing and dangerous, to those living and working in the regular routines and following socially accepted rules (Turner, 1974). To use Turner's (1974) terms, since new NPs are in an unclear and contradictory interstructural situation, they are apt to be perceived as being "contaminated" or impure, looked on as aberrations, disturbing, and even a threat to the status quo. As a result, they do not always have the support of their communities as they transition between roles. This only accentuates the experience of feeling disconnected.

The time of being adrift is also characterized as one of turbulence, "alternating emotions and perceptions with an overall range from easy to difficult and many in-betweens" (Heitz, Steiner, and Burman, 2004, p. 417). Waves of turbulence are commonly experienced by NPs as feelings of insecurity, disequilibrium, disorientation, anxiety, apprehension, and disorganization, along with the numerous and varied emotions that come with the loss of relationships, confidence, and control. One is immersed in an experience of feeling overwhelmed, inadequate, vulnerable, and confused — all emotions associated with being uncertain at a time when one experiences an intense awareness of being responsible for the protection of others. This uncertainty comes from the loss of previous reference points, abilities, and activities; the disruption of relationships and roles; incongruity between access and needs; discrepancies between what is anticipated or hoped for and what actually evolves; and having few or no NP role models. NPs' feelings of isolation and loneliness are thus heightened as a result of being disconnected — a time of waiting for that which is not yet known.

A situational change occurs when nurses move into the job titled "NP" and begin to engage in the new activities of performing detailed histories and physicals, making medical diagnoses, and prescribing treatments. However, the internal changes happen much more slowly. As a result, many NPs find themselves struggling in a kind of emotional abyss: they are not quite clear who they are or what is real. They experience emotional suffering and intense vulnerability as a result of taking on the characteristics of a persona that has no classification, for "it is as though they are being reduced or ground down to a uniform condition to be fashioned anew" (Turner, 1969, p. 95).

Perhaps one of Winslow Homer's most famous works, The Gulf Stream, helps to illustrate this time of being adrift. Painted in 1899, the canvas depicts a solitary man lashed to his boat, which is nested in a trough of waves. The mast and bowsprit have snapped, the tiller and rudder are gone, and a school of sharks circles the boat in blood-red water. On the horizon to the right, a looming storm presents a far more ominous outcome. Yet, if we look at Homer's painting more closely, the man appears to be strangely calm as he rests on his elbow, his mind seemingly alert as he searches for ways to manage the situation. On the horizon to the left, through the fog, there are both light and the silhouette of a ship under full sail: a possible rescue.

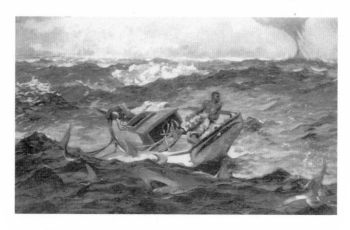

FIG. 1. Winslow Homer, *The Gulf Stream.* Courtesy of The Metropolitan Museum of Art.

Painful though it may be, the time when they are adrift offers NPs the best opportunity to be creative, develop into what they need and want to become, and renew themselves. As they struggle to stay afloat, a path opens to innovation and revitalization. It is thus both a dangerous and an opportune time, and is the very heart of the journey. NPs are introduced to new and special knowledge not previously accessible, and rapid and extensive learning and growth may occur. New NPs may begin to experience a transformation of identity, find new energy, and discover the fit for which they are searching. In being adrift, NPs have a perfect beginning for the process of transformation or metamorphosis, because being lost is just what is needed to properly prepare for the experience of being found.

The NPs' experiences of being disconnected, being uncertain, being lost, and struggling to stay afloat, all elements of being adrift, neither follow a linear pattern nor are necessarily limited to a single time in their journey. They experience these elements recursively, each weaving a unique design in the cocoon of change. In this respect, as well as being "a space in its own right"

(Froggatt, 1997, p. 125), transition is also a process of becoming, a mode of being. Being adrift may last for years, is not a single or simple initiation, and involves numerous experiences, each of which refines the outlook and lives of those engaged in the journey. The meanings attributed to this transitional experience are affected by such factors as the catalyst or call for the change, the individual's emotional and physical well-being, the individual's level of knowledge and skill preparation, the environmental resources and support, and the expectations of others who are themselves in transition. In fact, the NPs' transitional experiences are part of a matrix of transitions taking place simultaneously, such as the staff nurses' and medical colleagues' transition to accepting the presence of the NP, the nursing profession's transition to this advanced nursing practice role, and society's transition to this new health care provider. And finally, by its very nature, there is a mystery in what occurs during the hidden marginality or liminal state.

Being Disconnected

I am like a flag by far spaces surrounded.
I sense the winds that are coming, I must live them
while things down below are not yet moving;
the doors are still shutting gently, and in the chimneys is silence;
the windows are not yet trembling, and the dust is still heavy.

Then already I know the storms and am stirred like the sea.
And spread myself out and fall back into myself
and fling myself off and am all alone
in the great storm.

— Rainer Maria Rilke (1938), "Presentiment"

Although many NPs admit to having "horror stories about those nurses who eat their young," they hold great regard for their fellow nurses and speak about them and nursing with affection and loyalty. This is apparent in the jovial social atmosphere they describe as missing, particularly on nights and weekends, when there is a more relaxed and informal work environment. They miss the support that nurses give each other through difficult times. The change in their role brings about the loss of old ways of being that comes from working side by side, doing the same type of work, taking breaks together, and sharing stories in which there is a common sense of purpose and loyalties. "Being part of the team, but not really part of the team in terms of being at the bedside because they've flipped sides to giving orders" results in a sense of alienation. A special collegiality has been lost, and many NPs miss these previously taken-for-granted relationships. There is a sense of no longer belonging, a sense of loss of acceptance by the community of practice to whom they had once been strongly connected. With the realization that they have inevitably been changed in the process of becoming NPs, they also understand that this loss is permanent. Even if they should quit the NP role, a thought that often passes through their minds, the acquisition of new knowledge and skill means that they are no longer the nurses they once were.

> You go through separation, the letting go. I guess it's more like grieving for a secure position that you were in. And yet the challenge and the excitement and the opportunity of a new role still keeps you, has your appetite whetted with curiosity and wanting to develop those skills and have those learning opportunities. But at the same [time], it's a part of you that you were good at, and you are still good at, or I was still good at, but just along a different pathway. And it was sad to let go of it, to not be part of that team in the same sense of the intricacies. . . . Now you're always on the periphery.

Being disconnected is like being anchorless. As one NP reflected, in traditional bedside nursing shifts are structured around the to-do list of activities that are engrained in nurses' routines from the first days in clinical practicums. But in this new role, the NPs' sense of being disconnected is heightened by being uncertain about how to structure their days using the autonomy that they now have.

> The independent practice part of it was the biggest piece. . . . Going into a new role where — Oh, I don't have that anchor of having a patient assignment with specific tasks. What does that mean? There were no real roles and responsibilities written to clearly define — Okay, today I'm going to come on and every two hours you're going to do this, this and this. . . . It was fairly loose, and that independence and having to be responsible for my own autonomy and my self-learning activities was really new for me. So, trying to organize my day and people trusting me to be accountable for my hours. And so being given that autonomy wasn't something I was used to and so that autonomy piece was probably a bit of a transition.

Some NPs are instructed by nurse managers to refrain from wearing a uniform, answering bells, or helping other nurses in the giving of patient care so that the NP role can be differentiated from that of the traditional staff nurse. Despite their desire to demonstrate to nursing staff, patients, and families that they are both capable of and not above engaging in traditional nursing functions, some NPs see wisdom in this advice. Therefore, they disconnect themselves from familiar activities that provide them with some sense of purpose and meaning. Others remain engaged in these activities, recognizing that if there is an immediate patient need, then everyone should put their hands in the work that needs to be done. They feel that the priority must always be the patient, not what tasks are assigned to each person. Yet even they acknowledge the internal and external tension created when they realize that they must sometimes turn away from assisting nurses with hands-on patient care, turning instead to their own tasks, which are of equal importance and priority to patient well-being.

The simple fact that NPs spend the majority of their time interacting with staff physicians, fellows, and residents, eating, and socializing with them in the wee hours of the morning as they wait together for a new admission, may lead to the feeling that they are leaving the bedside nurse in the background. This loss of a sense of belonging to a community of nurses and the resulting grief that is experienced is palpable:

> I guess just to reconnect with nurses is part of what needs to be done. And I'm not sure what that means or how to do it exactly. I mean, we sometimes do these little education things and that helps, but there's more to it, and I'm not sure exactly what it is. But it's like you take a step up from bedside nursing if you will — I'm not sure that it's up, or if it's just over, I don't know — so you make this change, and you kind of just abandon nurses, maybe not nursing, but nurses. There has to be a way to integrate the two better. And we don't even eat in the nurses' lounge and I don't know what that means either, but it's just there. And nothing would happen if I stopped eating with the residents and ate with the nurses. No one would say anything. They might say, "Where were you at lunch?" And the nurses might kind of look at you but they wouldn't say anything either and they certainly probably wouldn't make me feel like I didn't belong there. But I have no idea if it would change their conversation at break time or not. I don't know if you're really so different that you would influence conversation or if you're really not that different in their eyes. . . . I miss it when it comes time to have their social things, and you're not sure if you should go or not.

How are NPs to re-establish their relationship with others in this new role? With whom are they to align themselves in a role frequently established as an "N of one" within their subspecialty practices? Wenger (1998) maintained that in order to do their job, individuals must align their activities and their interpretations of events with structures, forces, and purposes beyond their community of practice and so find their place in broader role processes. Yet during this time of being adrift, particularly because they are pioneers, NPs do not do this because structures are not yet known and understood, if indeed they are in place, and a sense of purpose has not yet been discovered. Turner (1974) suggested that individuals experiencing this in-between status tend to form a "community of passengers" in which they experience what he termed *communitas*, a spirit of comradeship and fellowship among those undergoing the same transition. But how can NPs develop or sustain the sense of "being in this together" when many of them are single passengers on the journey once they leave the educational setting?

There were two or three primary NPs in the hospital but again they were very busy and so it was hard to speak to similar events, or, it just wasn't the same. I don't know how you describe that, but it just would have been helpful to have had someone who's been there and done it before and knew exactly what you were experiencing. Because some days you'd go through it and you'd think, "Am I losing my mind? What am I doing here? . . . Everything is just all jumbled up [with] sort of that overwhelmingness and feeling so all alone.

If NPs work so frequently in isolation, can being disconnected be a transient, time-limited experience of passing from the centre of one cultural group to the centre of another? Or are NPs destined to find themselves in a more permanent marginalizing situation as a consequence of the context of their practice environment?

Perhaps the expression "I am afraid I'll miss the boat," commonly used by many NPs, takes on a new meaning when one considers that NPs are no longer "in the same boat" with others. This sense of being part of the team but not part of the team, "being in a place all of your own" that has no meaning, includes both the immediate care of the patient and a sense of not belonging to any group within the organization. One NP shared, "It's hard because you should be, from a clinical perspective, on the physicians' team, but they've got their own little intensivist team too. And so there's many teams in which you take part, but you're not always a part of. You're just a part of them when they think you should be a part. And so it's sort of like floating in your own little space." NPs experience a loss of identity since they are neither traditional nurses nor physicians.

NPs are also often unknown to each other, and thus feel disconnected from their own genre of nursing. One highly experienced NP lamented, "I still want to go and talk to someone, another NP. It's been something I've been wanting to do for a long time, to just work with another nurse practitioner for a week or so, because I never did work with anyone and I'm sure I could learn a lot about being a nurse practitioner." Most, even if they are not the only NP within their work setting, lack the time to invest in close relationships with their colleagues or to develop connections with others. Many work within institutions where the administration provides limited to no opportunities for NPs to get together, or they do not receive support from nursing management or their physician team so they can leave their clinical responsibilities in order to attend meetings. Nor do they have the energy to initiate a support group that can help them work through their feelings. A few join established local advanced nursing practice groups, most of which have been founded by CNSs. However, at this period in their professional development, there is virtually no connection between what they are experiencing in their clinical practice and what is being discussed. Again, they can find no sense of meaning or identity as NPs within a work structure in the course of their journey. The irony is that while they strive to carve a unique role that allows them to be more autonomous, more in control, and more connected, the very nature of these goals seems to highlight and heighten the experience of being disconnected.

As NPs describe the barriers to acceptance of their role, the relationship with physicians, nurses, and other health care providers inevitably surfaces as an issue. Support, encouragement, and assistance from professional colleagues are expectations learned from past experiences but not always present in this role, which results in the feelings of alienation, loneliness, vulnerability, anger, and frustration. Despite findings in the literature that have consistently identified lack of support as a problem (e.g., Brown and Draye, 2003; Heitz, Steiner, and Burnam, 2004), the degree of resistance and resentment, along with the depth of antagonism they experience from nurses, inevitably takes NPs by surprise. With alarming consistency, they describe senior staff who lacked care and concern for them, and who verbally abused them. How are identities shaped when NPs are forced to wrestle with the outright hostility that they encounter from some of their nursing colleagues as they try to begin to practise in their new role?

When bedside nurses challenge who they are and what they do in front of patients and families, or refuse to acknowledge the orders that they write, how does it affect their self-worth, the shaping of their identity, and their sense of being valued as NPs? One recounted, "And right in front of the patient she's like, 'So what do you think you are? Do you think you're better than everybody else around here? So if you think you're better than other nurses, is that why you're doing all this doctor stuff?'" Bedside nurses are in a central position to help NPs function more efficiently, but they can also undermine the NPs' confidence and effectiveness. When they do, they enhance the NPs' sense of being shunned by the clan and contribute to their experience of being disconnected, while prolonging the sense of being lost about who they actually are in this new role.

> *In the beginning some of [the nurses] were very rude. And I don't know if it was a sense of their being angry at someone else having the opportunity. I don't know if it's the "we–they" or I don't know what you would call it. It took about five years before the unit actually valued the role and had respect for its uniqueness. And some of it was a lack of understanding of what it was and the added skills opportunities and the implications of those. And so you'd have nurses in the unit saying, "Oh they always get everything. They're very specialized". . . . And so maybe that's just a felt need that you need to be valued in the position before you get that sense of security and ownership to a new role and the letting go of the old one.*

NPs readily admit that they come into the workplace unprepared to assume the full scope of the direct clinical practice component of the role, especially in the subspecialty for which they will be responsible. Key to the successful development of competence and confidence is the support and encouragement of physicians. Physicians, especially the staff physicians to whom they report for clinical management issues, are also essential in helping to establish their credibility with others. In the absence of NP role models and mentors, they are dependent on the close clinical supervision of the physicians who either lobbied for, or at least agreed to incorporate, the NP into the complement of professionals providing medical care to their patients. As they expend so much energy trying to master the knowledge base underlying the components traditionally identified as medical practice, NPs naturally lose sight of the science and art of nursing, a phenomenon described in research examining the family practices of primary health care NPs (see Anderson, Leonard, and Yates, 1974). NPs become obsessively task-oriented and this, for a period, becomes an end in itself. They describe being the physician's shadow for months or even several years. As they spend large amounts of time alongside physicians immersed in the diagnostic and therapeutic activities of medicine, their nursing identity is naturally submerged, further augmenting a sense of being disconnected.

But how can NPs who are "attached at the hip" to their medical colleagues feel so disconnected or marginalized from this group, even as they feel lucky enough to be fully supported by them? Why do they not become the centre of the physician's social environment? NPs are foreigners to the medical world; they are invited by some and denied entry by others. As such, they are positioned at its periphery, but being pioneers and lacking acute-care NP guides, they are unsure of the dimensions of the practice in which they are involved and therefore even have difficulties identifying its borders. Schultz (1971) captured this bind:

> He who wants to use a map successfully has first of all to know his standpoint in two respects: its location on the ground and its representation on the map. A foreigner has to face the fact that he lacks any status as a member of the social group he is about to join and is therefore unable to get a starting-point to take his bearings. He is, therefore, no longer permitted in considering himself as the centre of his social environment, and this fact causes again a dislocation of his contour lines of relevance. (p. 99)

NPs may feel disconnected from the medical group because they remain in a traditional one-down relationship with it. Anderson, Leonard, and Yates (1974) argued that without their own nursing base of information, philosophy of care, standards, and rationale, which have been temporarily set aside during this phase of learning, NPs are at the mercy of physicians, who, ultimately, remain in charge of patient care. As a result they cannot have a sense of truly being connected with their medical colleagues.

The social and political climate, both internal and external to the acute-care institution, continues to evolve and it remains unknown how this evolution will influence the presumed potential for movement between subordinate (nursing) and dominant (medical) worlds. This "not knowing" predicates an uncertain and unfixed acceptance of, and full functioning within, the confines of their world as NPs. For example, until recently, there was no legislation in Quebec that granted NPs the authority to write orders within acute-care institutions. In addition, the concept of medical directives, which facilitate at least some degree of autonomy in acute-care NP practice in Alberta and Ontario, does not exist in Quebec. Therefore, the majority of NPs in that province are able to assume little of their potential in their new role, and consequently increasing their sense that NPs are marginalized is sustained. Moreover, although they may be allowed to engage in some of the traditional functions of the medical cultural group, there is not an acknowledgment that they are, or will ever be, at its centre. Just as importantly, they do not want to be.

Most NPs describe at least a few episodes where physicians have been antagonistic and unwelcoming toward them. Worse yet, some reveal being consistently and blatantly ignored. Particularly frustrating are the occasions when NPs seek physician consultation but are refused or bypassed, making them feel invisible and ineffective. Physicians who fail to return their calls and surgeons or anaesthesiologists who state, "I cannot give my report to a nurse, I need to speak to the doctor to give the report" complicate the NPs' efforts at managing the patients' care. Some feel like second-class citizens when physicians do not attend medical rounds if an NP is scheduled to present, or NPs are refused admittance to resident teaching sessions even when the sessions concern their subspecialty service.

Certainly, under such circumstances, this part of the journey is experienced as chaotic, painful, and even traumatic. As a consequence, the sense of being disconnected and the accompanying feelings of vulnerability and alienation are even more accentuated and prolonged. This experience is made clear through an incident shared by an NP who, after two years in her current NP position and four years total as an NP, was only just beginning to feel a sense of belonging to the team:

> I didn't have any [specialty] background when I started but . . .
> they said, "Don't worry; we will provide this and this;" and
> I was promised some clinical mentorship from the physicians. . . .
> So when I get there, I'm in the operating room, I get paged for my
> first consult and I'm told by the person who's supposed to supervise
> or direct the inpatient care, "I'm really sorry but I don't review
> consults with you." And I said, "Well who's going to?" He said,
> "That's a very good question." So I was stuck. But I was so new,
> like I was just in a different world and a different language, it was
> really very different. And so for more than six months, I tried
> various strategies of helping myself learn. And I was unsuccessful.
> And then I went to my boss . . . and she said to me, "To learn,
> go to Dr. X's clinic." So I would go to the clinic and he would say,
> "Well I have a medical student and I have a resident and I only like
> two learners at a time." So I said, "Well, can I round with you?"
> Well, my office wasn't in the area and they would never call me.
> It was awful. . . . I had to do everything myself and sometimes
> the doors were really shut in my face. . . . I wasn't sleeping;
> I had to take more sick days in the first year of this job than I
> had in 22 years . . . but I was determined they wouldn't break me.

The necessary focus of the NPs' learning at this point is the medical agenda, as they are kept busy clinically learning how to independently apply the knowledge and skill learned in school. As a result of this intense and narrow focus, they have no time to be present with the patients and families. The search for being more connected in their nursing practice seems more distant and elusive than it had ever been in their traditional nursing roles. "I just don't have enough time; I'm ordering the pills and I'm doing the spinal, while the nurses are talking to the mom, teaching her how to give the Septra and comforting the child," said one NP. "I miss bedside nursing; I want to be on the other side of the fence and be that comforting person at the bedside again." The resulting turbulence leaves them questioning their choice and reminiscing about what they have left behind.

Feelings of marginality and lack of connection are also a direct consequence of frequently being involved in defensive encounters with colleagues, patients, and patients' families: "Are you my resident today?" "Well, you're ordering things; you're prescribing things; you're diagnosing. Look at the number of years you've spent in school with your master's. Why didn't you go through to be a doctor?" How does one retain a sense of connectedness to nursing when nurses identify the NP role as belonging to medicine?

Being Uncertain

[A]nd while I supposed myself to be looking as salt as Neptune himself, I was, no doubt, known for a landsman by every one on board as soon as I hove in sight. . . . In a short time . . . we began to heave up the anchor. I could take but little part in all these preparations. My little knowledge of a vessel was at fault. Unintelligible orders were so rapidly given and so immediately executed; there was such a hurrying about, and such an intermingling of strange cries and stranger actions, that I was completely bewildered. There is not so helpless and pitiable an object in the world as a landsman beginning a sailor's life. (Dana, 2001, pp. 6–8)

Acute-care NPs provide care to patients with complex, acute, and often life-threatening health problems. Hemodynamic instability, pulmonary compromise, and nosocomial infections are frequent concerns. Many hospitalized patients have multisystem diseases, which can contribute to atypical presentations of symptoms. Acute complications of chronic illnesses can develop in response to therapeutic treatments for other conditions (e.g., an acute exacerbation of congestive heart failure after a blood transfusion). The complexity of health problems is compounded by therapeutic interventions or technologic modalities, many of which obscure important physical assessment findings. The risks associated with the physiologic instability of patients and the potential for life-threatening complications often require NPs to make rapid clinical judgments in tense situations. Data may be simultaneously overwhelming and incomplete. These factors challenge the diagnostic reasoning process, potentially impeding hypothesis generation and evaluation, problem identification, and treatment decision-making. Yet NPs, like physicians, are tasked with the job of accurately diagnosing and treating their patients' health problems. They may doubt their abilities to use what they know in order to care for patients safely, and be concerned they should know more than what they have been taught. This creates the experience of being uncertain, a sense of being overwhelmed, as they continue to learn from the ground level up how to attack patient-care management on top of learning to master the procedural skills required in their practice.

I wondered at the expectations. I wondered at the other NPs who do it and do they think they're doctors and I wondered if I had the skills or the knowledge to do it. I wondered if I'd make a fool of myself. I'd always given someone the information and just done what they told me to do. Well now I was going to be the teller and that's so much responsibility and it was just so scary thinking that one day maybe I would make a decision that would be harmful or wrong. It was just so very overwhelming. Very scary.

Suzanne Gordon (2005, p. 10) observed that within a traditional health care model the physician is seen as "the captain of the medical ship" in the acute-care setting. The charted course regarding the daily medical plan of patient care is handed down in the form of orders that nurses are expected to carry out. In the NP role, one is in the position of performing in the "captain" capacity. However, NPs do so without a navigational chart or dedicated guide familiar with the NP journey. This leaves them in the position in which most pioneers find themselves: thrilled and exhilarated about the potential opportunities for autonomy and intellectual challenge, but also shocked and overwhelmed with what they do not know, with few institutional supports to assist them with integration into their new practices.

NPs are persistently made aware of their uncertainty by the stressful thoughts and feelings rooted in their day-to-day consciousness as they engage in the new activities of their practice. Some NPs describe being uncertain as merely unsettling. However, most admit to feeling terrified, being scared, and being frightened; feelings that are present to some degree most, if not all, of the time and then heightened each time they are required to perform something new.

It was very frightening at the beginning. For my first two years, every time I had a call to come see something the one thing I used to do when I got woken out of bed was say, "Dear God help me make it through the night." Seriously! "Help me make the right decision." People are lying if they don't tell you they're scared for those first two years.

For many months, or as long as two to three years, NPs can live with the uncomfortable awareness that they may make a mistake that could cause a patient's death. Not knowing if the outcomes of their decision-making will be the right ones creates a disequilibrium born of fear for the patient's safety. Many NPs are preoccupied with "terrible things you just can't imagine," particularly after they leave the clinical area and have quiet time to dwell upon the daily course of events. Even after two years of experience, one NP described that at the end of each day she still lived with niggling doubts that she may have missed something. Faye Ferguson (1991) gave insight into this experience of being uncertain: "When faced with uncertainty . . . the emotions can easily hold sway, carrying one away with thoughts of disaster. During these moments or hours one feels trapped, captive to the terror of what might be possible." (p. 316)

A certain gravity is associated with being uncertain that is expressed as mental turmoil. Each decision feels like a narrow escape from causing a deadly outcome. Treading water and barely keeping afloat, while trying to keep their "heads above water, trying not to kill anyone, and trying just to get comfortable," creates an overall state of exhaustion, the result of constantly being mentally on guard and second guessing oneself. One NP recalled that for nearly three years she worked frantically to absorb as much academic knowledge as she could while attempting to make it have practical meaning in her decision-making with each new patient. An inability to sleep and having nightmares or dreaming all night long about their patients are common issues:

One of my fears is that I will write an order and it will be misread
or incorrectly processed or something and then something harmful
could happen. . . . The first time I wrote an order I shook for
probably a day. . . . Again the mental turmoil is [that] I spend a
lot of my time after work more or less just going through my head
the events of the day. . . . But I always look at — What have I
done? What have I ordered? Was there something better? Should
I have done it differently? . . . So there have been a few times when
I've actually gotten home and I've had to turn around and come
back because I've second-guessed myself. And it's been silly, but
I've needed to do that in order to put my mind at ease.

NPS' mental fatigue is compounded by the drain of energy required
to hide their inner turmoil. In the following passage, an NP
describes the heaviness, or gravity, of being uncertain. This passage was delivered in a tone that invoked the arduousness and
tiring nature of not knowing.

I was very tired. I was so tired from making decisions. I just
remember thinking I don't want to make another decision today
about anything. And it was such hard work, such hard work to do
this. And you know — Lasix q6, q8, q12? I don't know. Once a
day? You've got to think about this, this, this, and this. You need
to look at a weight gain, and fluids, fluid balance, urine output.
And it was just so tiring because there was so much to think about.
I can remember going home after these 24-hour-call shifts, and
not [being] physically tired from being up, but just mentally tired
from having to make these decisions.

Questions, rather than answers, dominate. Do I have the ability to
make the decisions? How should I approach this problem? How do I solve it? Do
I know what to do? What do others want me to know and do versus what do I
need to know and do? Similar to Benner's (1984) nurse as the advanced

beginner, NPs are uncertain about the tension between what they perceive they know and what they should but do not yet know. Fearing they will never make or be capable of making accurate clinical management decisions, will never be able to carry the weight of responsibility that results from making those decisions or understand the expectations required of them, the milestones to be met, and whether others will be there to support them — these are all elements in their uncertainty.

NPs also fear that poor decision-making will negatively impact NPs' professional reputation, and they report that the burden of reputation protection is heavy. They must not only protect their own professional reputation but also the reputations of physicians associated with them. Ultimately, each believes that the reputation of the whole acute-care NP movement is in her or his hands — a finding also reported in Buehler's (1987) research with primary-care NPs. This is reflected in one NP's comments:

> I mean, you're always afraid that you're going to screw up and
> be caught screwing up. And there is this onus on new practitioners
> because in this province and in this city nurse practitioners are new;
> like three years is about it where I work. So there's always this
> onus that you don't want it to be, "Oh, those nurse practitioners!"
> You don't want that ever to be heard. You want to provide excellence
> all the time. Of course that's not realistic though. . . . You work so
> hard to gain credibility and gain trust and be taken seriously, that
> you don't want to do something stupid, because one little thing can
> undo so much hard work.

Living with a persistent sense of uncertainty about their abilities to engage in a new level of decision-making is linked with not knowing how to think like a physician. Yet from the time that they walk into the clinical setting, they are required to make numerous and varied medical decisions and provide safe care for patients:

When I first started I had a lot of on-the-job learning to do, even though I went through the NP program. It was great but there were a lot of knowledge gaps . . . things like how to manage a diabetic patient for instance; or, though we had microbiology and that kind of stuff and prescription of antibiotics, when you actually get into the clinical area and you're dealing with infections and organisms and sensitivities and antibiotics and this whole thing with resistance, there's a huge learning curve to that. And then more critical-care stuff, stuff like gut ischemia and oesophageal varices and bleeding ulcers and peritonitis and pancreatitis and adrenal insufficiency and it just goes on and on and stuff that I didn't know and I'm like, "Oh my God." Like here I am in this critical-care environment and look at all this stuff, and I'm like "Ahhh!!" And what if I compromise all these vulnerable patients?

Acute-care NPs understand that the "NP part" of their job requires a form of medical apprenticeship in the first several years in order to learn clinical management of patients in their specialty population. But despite whether it is what they expected or wanted, for a number of months they suddenly find themselves unsure of what to do because, as nurses, they have "not been trained to think the way doctors do. It's a whole different way of thinking and it's really hard." Although they have a sense that there should be more to the NP role than being a physician replacement, that is exactly what they do during the apprenticeship period. Many of them mention that they function from a medical model instead of a nursing model of care but, in hindsight, realize this is necessary at the beginning — an understanding that has also been noted in the primary-care NP literature (Kelly and Mathews, 2001).

One of the characteristics of belonging to a homogeneous community of practice is the development of a shared culture. Wenger (1998, p. 83) noted that the culture of a community of practice includes routines, words, tools, ways of doing things, stories, gestures, symbols, actions, or concepts that the community has produced or adopted and which have become part of its practice. It also includes the discourse by which members create meaningful statements about the world and the styles by which they express their forms of membership and their identities as members. Acute-care NPs, however, as pioneers in their practice and as people frequently working in isolation from other NPs, usually have no community of practice through which to experience their world and find meaningful engagement related to their role. Nor has the wider Canadian acute-care NP community of practice yet been able to establish a historically recognizable culture such that everyone knows what NPs are to be doing. In other words, other communities of practice such as nursing, medicine, and pharmacy do not yet know, appreciate, and therefore trust who NPs are and what they can do. As one acute-care NP commented, NPs are thus required "to prove [they are] legitimate in providing care, because until others understand the NP role and have insight into our training, [NPs] will always be compared to other physicians, other residents; whereas if they came up to them as a medical resident and I'm X year, then they have a certain conception of what that person should be capable of doing, what they have been exposed to or not exposed to."

Initially, then, the negotiation of meaning for NPs is created primarily in their social relationships with physicians, on whom they are reliant for the delivery of safe practice, along with the nurses with whom they work. Yet, once they enter clinical practice, NPs find themselves on the fringes of medicine's community of practice, of which they have limited knowledge and know-how. In order to belong to communities of practice, they must engage in the practices, routines, language, and conventions of those communities. In other words, they need to do whatever it takes to make mutual engagement possible. This means that they must demonstrate that they know how to think like the members of a given community. Yet, not knowing how to think like a physician is partially the root of their uncertainty, because not knowing how to think like a physician is to some extent a measure of not yet knowing enough of the language of a physician.

Words that aren't my own
Language foreign to my mind
I'm spinning my wheels.

— **Mika Yoshimoto** (2008, p. 22)

NPs simply do not at first have the depth and breadth of terminology that is associated with advanced anatomical, physiological, pathophysiological, and pharmacological knowledge. Not knowing the language results in either not understanding others or not being understood by others. Mutual engagement is impeded and the feeling of being uncertain intensifies.

Understanding how distressful uncertainty can be, and understanding the tendency for uncertainty to diminish a person in his or her own eyes despite the previous level of confidence and competence, is revealed in the manner in which this NP expresses the experience of not knowing.

It is hard because you don't know if you're on the same page. And when I think of describing an X-ray to somebody — because even to this day you can say, "Well, he has that kind of blah, blah, blah" — but they don't necessarily use the same words that can mean the same thing. And X-rays are quite hard, because there's something there and they want to know what it is. Well, I think it's this because I see a shadow, and you don't call it lucency or darkness, or it's fluffy. And I know them better now, but at the time — near the heart, near the thymus or the hilum. They ask you so you end up saying, "Well, I'm not sure that I see that or not. I can't tell you."

In fact, learning to speak with the physicians' terminology is what makes mutual engagement with the medical discipline possible. Physicians' speech is associated with the way in which text is formatted and presented, the way in which information is edited, so that it is orally represented to the medical audience in a manner they accept and appreciate:

> The type of information that physicians want to hear is not the same as what nurses want to hear. . . . I remember when I was a novice NP, I would report everything in tremendous detail and the comments were frequently, "This is very thorough but I don't need this. As a nurse I can understand that you would want to know these things, but from a physician's perspective this is not what I'm interested in." And the difference was learning that when you're talking to physicians to communicate what they want to know, and in that way you communicate that you understand what's important to them.

Being uncertain with regard to their use of medical language and speech becomes critical in relation to such actions and artifacts as medical rounds, the order sheet, physician notes, and discharge summary records. Although nurses are familiar with and have shared points of reference regarding such traditions, these traditions do not impose the same meaning when viewed from a bedside nurse's perspective as when viewed from the perspective of being a new NP. The particular nature of nursing's understanding of these elements of practice lies in the rules and regulations, or structures, applied to these artifacts and conventions, which are determined as much from within nursing as from without.

In his classic work *Truth and Method*, Gadamer (1989) interpreted the concept of *play* (both literal and metaphorical). He reasoned that play has its own essence in the fact that it becomes an experience that changes the person who experiences it, "independent of the consciousness of those who play" (Gadamer, 1989, p. 102). Gadamer's interpretation helps us to understand that, once nurses make the choice to play as NPs, they expressly separate this new playing behaviour from their other nursing behaviours thereby indicating they are "choosing to play this game rather than that" (Gadamer, 1989, p. 107). They must learn to play anew in the game's designated spaces: "The space in which the game's movement takes place is not simply the open space in which one 'plays oneself out,' but one that is specially marked out and reserved for the movement of the game" (Gadamer, 1989, p. 107). NPs must learn to carry themselves with a certain type of comportment, inclusive of both linguistic and non-linguistic genres, and to use the predetermined choreography between players:

> That all play is playing something is true here, where the ordered to-and-fro movement of the game is determined as one kind of *comportment* among others . . . even if the proper essence of the game consists in his disburdening himself of the tension he feels in the purposive comportment. (Gadamer, 1989, p. 103)

Gadamer demonstrates that in successfully performing the tasks of the game, "one is in fact playing oneself out. The self-presentation of the game involves the player's achieving, as it were, his own self-presentation by playing — i.e., presenting — something" (Gadamer, 1989, p. 108).

Now previously known linguistic and non-linguistic elements take on new interpretations when used to new effect by the NP and viewed from a new trajectory. For instance, NPs describe medical rounds, a quintessential medical play, as a stage where they are now players who are placed front and centre without the requisite skills to stand upright and not feel exposed. In this once familiar but now unfamiliar metaphorical playground, NPs constantly experience uncertainty due to not knowing what to expect, how to articulate the limited knowledge they have, and what level of knowledge is expected of them. During medical rounds, they have a sense of no longer possessing the protection of being a spectator but being required to actively perform without the requisite tools:

> It was like having to go into an exam every morning [with] no idea what the exam would be on. Furthermore, it's an exam in front of ten other people and they'll all know what you know and don't know, and that was very stressful. . . . And because you would get quizzed on rounds, everyone's watching and listening. . . . And we are treated very much like a resident and so then you're asked why this and why that and what do you know about this and what do you know about that and tell me about this or that. So, I mean, I haven't been to medical school; half that stuff I've never heard of, and all of a sudden I'm expected to know it. It's quite daunting.

Acute-care NPs appreciate from their years of working in acute-care teaching institutions that medical rounds are part of medicine's initiation process. Rounds are, in Turner's terms (1969), a rite of passage, part of the ritual process created by the medical community of practice to assist in the transition from one place, state, and social position to another. In this milieu, others, particularly physicians, actually judge NPs against their definition of competent NP performance, a definition that mimics their own particularistic philosophy of medical practice. NPs understand that it is within their capabilities to articulate their understanding and summarize the plan of care such that members of the team will develop a respect for their abilities, the NP role, and themselves as individuals. Being uncertain in this milieu brings about a strong awareness that "everyone is judging you." NPs feel that perhaps others are seeing them for the very first time in terms of what they are lacking, not for the competent or expert nurses they had been previously. What really makes being uncertain so discomforting is the constant awareness of one's deficiencies that this visibility and awareness of uncertainty invokes.

Similarly, NPs are required to engage in medical discourse using the written format within medical artifacts. However, not knowing how to write medical orders, medical progress notes, and discharge summaries adds to NPs' feelings of uncertainty, which are further intensified by the uncertainty that comes with crossing boundaries to spaces that had been previously forbidden to them as nurses:

> So having to learn the language and really not being given any course on how to write an order per se, and there is a format on how to write orders, what needs to be included; there is a process around that. And that isn't part of the orientation or internship or whatever it is called. And there needs to be more value put on it because the significance of that is huge, and it was an area where I didn't have any experience with it.

New NPs are also unsure of how to interpret information in a new and different way, which culminates in generating a possible problem list, a differential diagnosis, and a treatment plan. Not knowing how to make a diagnosis or whether it is the right one is frightening, sometimes even paralyzing, and this is only accentuated when new NPs have limited knowledge and experience within their specialty area, precluding them from identifying patterns. Not knowing routines and what the various doctors in their practice want and will accept compounds their feelings of uncertainty. They immediately realize that knowing how to make a differential diagnosis is not something learned in nursing, and it is a concept that can be quite difficult to grasp. Learning to think of all the possibilities, particularly when one has limited knowledge, while at the same time being able to prioritize a plan around the most likely possibility when scant information is available, is like climbing the mast of a ship without a safety line:

> Making the diagnosis is difficult at times. I personally struggle with it unless it's fairly obvious. I never have done very well pulling differential diagnoses out of the hat and I think that's where I need to do a bit more. . . . We get a lot of our patients from Emergency and they've got the diagnosis down in front of us. So I look at the diagnosis and I think, "Why did he choose that? Well alright, belly pain. Oh my God, there's probably a gazillion things that cause belly pain". . . but if I have to see somebody cold turkey that's where I struggle a bit. We can diagnose congestive heart failure easily; if you come in with high sugars, well you're obviously in a diabetic state. It's the not-so-clear cases — I'm thinking, well, some guy's diagnosed dengue fever; where did that come from? Why did he diagnose that? Well, I'm not familiar with the pattern of that; that doesn't even pop into my mind. And then again, I think, "Well goodness, should I know that?" And then this self-doubt thing overcomes me: "Well, my God, I wouldn't have written down dengue fever." So that's what goes through my mind.

Even when they are able to make the diagnosis accurately, verbalizing or writing the diagnosis can be overwhelming in and of itself, as it too is a boundary not previously crossed:

> I guess one of the things that stunned me the most and took me a long time to get over was being able to actually write that the man

had a nose bleed rather than saying the man had blood coming from his nose; so that as an NP I can actually diagnose that nose bleed. So the hardest thing to get my mind around was now I could suddenly do these things that you were always told you couldn't.

Buehler (1987, p. 50) wrote, "Educators and physicians repeatedly point out that the single most important attribute of an NP is [their] 'knowing and practicing within [their] limits.' The clinical judgments that they make determine how others evaluate their compliance with this norm." Yet, the fact that what they are questioning is beyond their scope of practice reveals the NPs' struggle to determine the set of expectations about the level of knowledge and skill required within their practices. The acute-care NPs' uncertainty is accentuated because there is not yet an aggregate of NPs performing the same role within the same context, except, perhaps, in the field of neonatal nursing. There has been no historical determination of what exactly they do, how they are to do it, and the level to which they are to perform it. Ironically, they cannot discover independence within their practice until they know their limitations — limitations that are defined by their scope of practice.

For NPs, worrying is a common response to living with uncertainty. They feel a sense of dread about "the worst thing you can imagine happening," which looms over them until it does happen. They worry about whether they will be able to independently reproduce the decision-making sequence without missing critical steps. Have they gathered all the information necessary to make an accurate diagnosis and treatment plan? Can they successfully repeat what they do, such as performing a psychomotor skill under pressure or in a different circumstance?

Worrying is also associated with the desire to do what is right and to do what is good for the patients entrusted to their care. Acute-care NPs carry a mature and practised understanding of what it means for the patient and family to provide (or fail to provide) the "right" treatment. Knowing how to provide the right care is essential to clinical judgment and ethical comportment. Central to their feeling adrift is concern about being able — or unable — to respond to patients' physiological needs, protecting them in their physical vulnerability and helping them to feel safe in the NP's hands. Typically, there is a sense of hyper-alertness and hyper-responsibility, and NPs deliberately engage multiple coping mechanisms. In contrast to Benner's (1984) findings, this sense of hyper-responsibility is present in the initial part of the NPs' journey, not at the competent stage of the novice-to-expert continuum. This may be because they know what it means to be competent nurses and therefore understand the tensions and competing risks involved in managing various clinical situations. In addition, as experienced nurses they have long lost their naivety about the absolute trustworthiness of the environment and the legitimacy of co-workers' knowledge. Benner noted that naivety normally allows the beginning learner to absorb information as fact and truth, and for this reason they experience a sense of certainty about the outcomes of their actions, along with an excitement about learning. Yet for many NPs, this sense of fun and exhilaration is not experienced until later in their journey.

NPs readily acknowledge that as experienced bedside nurses they believed they had the experiential knowledge to determine what treatment was required in the clinical situation, although they did not possess the authority to act upon it. Yet ironically, when permission is finally granted for them to act upon their knowledge and skill, they immediately realize that being *able* to do what needs to be done involves much more than being *permitted* to use advanced theoretical and experiential knowledge. One NP noted, "When you actually have that accountability or decision-making or responsibility for the decisions, it becomes much different than just suggesting, 'What do you think about _____?'" With the granting of authority to diagnose, prescribe, and treat in ways previously denied them, NPs must not only acknowledge that they may and can do what needs to be done for patients, but also acknowledge and accept responsibility for it. Ironically, they may now experience a lack of self-confidence and hesitation as a consequence of being faced with increased responsibility and accountability for the patient's health, which results in uncertainty.

Why is the NPs' relationship with responsibility so personal and intense? Is it possible that having been an expert nurse, with a high degree of knowledge and skill embedded in a strong sense of moral responsibility, only serves to heighten the tension and apprehension around issues of responsibility and their consequences? Throughout the course of their careers, they have seen the negative outcomes of errors in clinical judgment. They are also imbued with a strong nursing ethos that emphasizes moral and ethical standards, a duty to practise informed by an ideology of "conscientiousness" and a "high ethical and professional standard" of care (see Nightingale, 1992, p. 3). It is an ideology that emphasizes caring for those with illness rather than curing illness. Therefore, NPs experience an internal angst that may arise from a clash between their own values and expectations of self and the "what if" consequences of those expectations when they engage in acts associated with curing illness.

NPs are not originally educated within an ideology that facilitates objectification of the patient as a diseased entity or a bodily part that requires repair or cure. Rather, they have been indoctrinated in a caring philosophy that asks them to react "responsively and responsibly" (van Manen, 1991, p. 97) to the call of the vulnerable. Yet they now find themselves engaging in risk-taking, seemingly in direct opposition to this very call. To take risks, which is what is demanded in situations of informational ambiguity as

it is applied to medicine (Haas and Shaffir, 1987), is a characteristic that neither comes naturally nor has been learned through
their previous training as nurses. In fact, as one NP noted about
the mindset associated with risk-taking and its application to clinical decision-making, "I think that's a difference between nursing
and medicine: medicine is sort of 'the buck stops here,' where
for a lot of nursing practice it's 'call the physician.'" Subsequently,
because of uncertainty, NPs worry and experience premature guilt
for what might occur if the "what if" situations comes to pass.

"Being-guilty," Heidegger (1962) wrote, "has the significa-
tion of 'being responsible for' [schuld sein an] — that is, being the
cause or author of something, or even 'being the occasion' for
something," and "'being-guilty' as 'having debts' [schulden haben]
is a way of Being with Others in the field of concern, as in providing something or bringing it along" (p. 327). These two ways
of "being-guilty," when experienced in combination, define a
kind of behaviour that Heidegger (1962) called "making oneself
responsible" (p. 327), which he argued results from one person
"having the responsibility for the Other's becoming endangered"
(p. 327). "Being-guilty" in this sense results from "the breach of
a 'moral requirement'" (Heidegger, 1962, p. 328), even if that
breach is only an anticipated one.

Thus we may say that NPs experience intense feelings of vulnerability embedded in feelings of future-oriented culpability
concerning their clinical decision-making when they realize that
they could inflict harm upon the Other. For French philosopher
Emmanuel Levinas (1996, p. 131), the face is a mode in which the
vulnerable Other is revealed, and we recognize that we have been
summoned to responsibility: "The Other becomes my neighbour
precisely through the way the face summons me, calls for me, begs
for me, and in so doing recalls my responsibility, and calls me into
question." Levinas acknowledged that in this ethical imperative,
responsibility to Other "goes beyond what I may or may not have

done to the Other or whatever acts I may or may not have committed" (Levinas, 1996, p. 131). Thus, the emotional and mental unease NPs experience in being uncertain can be seen to result from the moral imperative to be vigilant in the face of the Other.

As most NPs are quick to point out, learning to write physician orders and fill in the physician order sheet causes them trepidation. They come face to face with the weight of the responsibility that they carry in the act of writing. On one level, the writing of medical orders on the doctor's order sheet, medical progress notes in the physician's section, and the discharge note, along with their signature, are clear examples of the operation of micropower. Yet at the same time, this writing carries heavy symbolism and strong structural connections to explicit, hierarchical power structures:

> We write orders all the time as nurses but we take verbal orders and we just transcribe them. . . . The first time I wrote an order, I have to say, it was somewhat exhilarating. . . . And once you get over that, the responsibility part of your brain kicks in and . . . again you need to think through your orders, and think through your decisions as to why you are ordering something, and what you're going to do with that information once you've ordered it. . . . So it was very exciting . . . to have this little power that we have, but again there's a lot of responsibility with that, which again, I take quite seriously when I'm writing those orders.

However, at another level, the writing of orders and the transcribing of thought processes in progress notes is about the NPs' willingness to accept responsibility for setting into motion a series of cause-and-effect activities and simultaneously appreciating the gravity of those actions. One NP said, "Always in the back of my mind is that the pen is the mightiest thing. You know, you must always be very careful with what you're writing because with a pen stroke, you could harm someone." The writing of an order and the use of the pen, once a taken-for-granted activity with a taken-for-granted tool, now takes on new significance; pen put to paper has become a potential weapon, and NPs wield the instrument of potential harm, even destruction:

> I guess the biggest adjustment . . . was the writing of the orders
> on the order sheet. It was a real funny feeling . . . that physician
> territory of physician order sheet and a nurse writing on the
> physician order sheet. It seems so silly. But anyway, I mean . . .
> it seems so legal and liable and it was interesting. And you didn't
> want to make an error because it was in copies and when you see
> it in [a] court of law years down the road, and you recognize your
> writing on that physician sheet, you realize just how significant it is.

This power of the pen has also been described in Richard Peschel's recollection of a haunting incident from his medical residency in his story "The Ritual and the Death Certificate." This story appears in a remarkable book, *When a Doctor Hates a Patient and Other Chapters in a Young Physician's Life* (Peschel and Peschel, 1986). In this story, Peschel described the first time he had to pronounce a patient dead. Having held the stethoscope to the patient's chest listening for some sounds of breathing and a heartbeat, and having "stood around for a while so it would appear that [he] had spent a respectable amount of time determining that the patient was dead," (Peschel and Peschel, 1986, p. 71) he felt "somehow disappointed" (p. 71) in the whole process. In other words, Peschel had found there was "little reflection about a human life having just ended" (Peschel and Peschel, 1986, p. 71) However, when he went to complete the death certificate, and was instructed that he must use "the Brady pen" (p. 72) — Brady being the name of the morgue — he was suddenly confronted with the gravity of the responsibility he carried.

Prior to taking on the NP role, when nurses use pens and physician order sheets, they have no need for focal awareness of themselves and these tools. The skills and practices that they bring to the activity are so familiar to them that they are simply unaware of their existence. However, when they become NPs, they encounter the pen and order sheet in a way that brings about a state of unease. As a result, they have an opportunity to reflect, detaching themselves from ongoing practical involvement in the project of writing orders and progress notes, to better understand the significance of what they do when engaged in these activities. The resulting stepping back from "I" and the recognition of "I" in this situation creates not only self-reflection but also self-conflict. *What is the meaning of all this? Who am I? Am I becoming alienated from myself as a nurse and from nursing as part of my world by engaging in these acts of writing orders or making these types of clinical decisions?* But perhaps, just as Heidegger (1962, pp. 293–301) philosophically argued about the experience of worry and responsibility, NPs are uncomfortable with every role they can play in the world of health care during the period of being adrift, because in the act of acknowledging they may cause the death of an Other, they have to face their own mortality. Simply stated, NPs find themselves being forced to realize the importance of choosing a possibility and defining themselves by it.

The NPs' sense of responsibility to the Other is not limited only to the patient. However, when NPs refer to the level of responsibility that they carry, they are not referring to a hierarchical level, which would then have a tendency to diminish or denigrate the responsibility that staff nurses bear. Rather, the level of responsibility speaks to a different sphere of influence and the layers of responsibility that NPs bear, which are different from and broader than those of the traditional bedside nursing role. When NPs write orders that will be carried out by others, they are responsible for being the clinical authority on medical management issues, and they know that the health care professionals who carry out their orders "take on some degree of faith" that they are correct. The impact or consequence of a wrong diagnosis or treatment may not only result in a negative outcome for the patient but also may compromise the emotional and professional integrity of all the health care providers involved.

Joan Cassell's (1992) study of the work of surgeons provides further insight into NPs' experience of being uncertain as it relates to the new sense of responsibility that they carry. The outcomes of their actions are *attributable*; that is, the NP and the patient, the family, and the team know the NP is responsible when events go well or poorly. Also, as noted earlier, much of their work is now more visible; their actions take place before a public composed of the patient and family, nurses, and often the staff physician, residents, and other physician subspecialists, all of whom admire success and note failure. The NP's every move is now more closely scrutinized and publicly judged. "Marjorie," a critical care nurse, described the shame she felt when she accidentally cut an umbilical artery catheter instead of the venous one she was attempting to replace. Although she had requested that a vascular surgeon be paged to assist her with its retrieval, "half the hospital" responded to the *stat* call that had been placed, a request the NP had not made:

And my face was burning; I felt like I didn't want to be there anymore but I kind of coped until I was thinking — God, how am I going to tell these parents? They weren't there, so that was better. If they had been there I would have had to explain how all these people had to get involved and what needed to happen to do [retrieve the catheter] and I would have been much more mortified.

Being Lost

One day you leave, you go to school, and the next day when you
come back you're a different person because you do something else
different. . . . It's the same place, I'm the same person, but I don't
know anything anymore, because finishing school you don't pretend
that you know the role very well. . . . I'm physically the same person.
I didn't change. I could be of some help to nurses but in a different way,
but nobody, including me, knows exactly what I can do or what I'm
allowed to do. And so I'm different, yes and no. But who am I? I mean
I knew I was a nurse, but maybe I was trending toward the medical
model at the time . . . and you just don't know who you are anymore.

Being lost is the experience of a loss of identity; NPs are unsure of
how to respond to such questions as *Who are you?*, *Are you a nurse or a
resident?*, or *Where do you belong?* Instead, these questions are answered
by asking more questions. The constant focus on the instrumental
nature of their role leads them to wonder: *Is this what being an NP
is all about? Could it be that I am a physician substitute? Where is the nurse in
the NP role? Is this what I really want? Should I quit?* These types of questions suggest that NPs experience disillusionment during this initial
period. Disillusionment is the internal perception created by role
realities, and, as noted by Heitz, Steiner, and Burman (2004) in
their work on role transition, it leads to self-questioning of why
one endures the role, given the internal and external challenges.
NPs say it is difficult to adhere to the ideals of holistic care and
health promotion while responding to the various expectations
of self and others, none of which may even seem attainable. They
articulate a constant struggle with holding on to who they were
and what they did, in the face of who they are becoming as a result
of what they are now doing. Because of the situational pressures,
they often feel it is difficult to hold to the NP ideals and establish
a role that is different from that of physicians.

Even the familiar world of nursing is now far off and inaccessible. Many NPs do not realize how loyal to nursing they are until they are away from their "home." As a result, they become more aware of what belonging to the community of nursing means to them, because now a sense of belonging is re-experienced in a different way, more like being "a drop of oil on the water" (Wu, 1991, p. 274). Zhou Wu (1991) addresses analogous feelings in his writing on the lived experience of language learning and acculturation:

> The meaning of the old world . . . is often elusive. It is very hard to measure its volume. This body of water in the heart of a foreigner can be as vast as an ocean, as it often occupies his or her whole inner world. . . . I am homesick, but I don't know what I am missing. (p. 274)

Feeling like an impostor or fraud is a common experience for new acute-care NPs: "For nearly a year I felt like I didn't belong here; this wasn't home; this wasn't welcoming and I was an impostor in my role." An inability to articulate what they do and how to do it, rather than "this is where I can be found throughout the week," contributes to this sense of homelessness and lack of self. Feeling like an impostor is also an experience born out of being uncertain. NPs feel as if they are trying to pass themselves off as insiders while being outsiders to a special group of people who all have qualities or traits that they do not. They are plagued with nagging self-doubt and a fear that their colleagues will realize that they are not "one of them."

On the one hand, as NPs experience being disconnected, they may feel that they are nurse impostors because they no longer belong to nursing. On the other hand, by the very nature of working on the margins of the medical community of practice, particularly during the time of being uncertain, they may feel like physician impostors. As a result, they may feel that they are not who they should be and are somehow falling short of the expectations and standards for someone in the physician's position. And yet this is not quite true either, for they know that they are not physicians, even though they need to have some of the same knowledge and skills.

Perhaps NPs do not fail to measure up to the ideal of what they are supposed to be; rather, they fail to see who they truly are. NPs qualify for the positions they occupy and are deemed competent at what they do for the level of experience they have attained, as signified by a licence to practice. But part of feeling like an impostor is the belief that everyone else fits the ideal except them. A few compare themselves to other NPs whom they have seen in action during their educational experience, or to other NPs within their own practice setting. Others have created their expectations for the NP role based on a combination of the discourse (e.g., NPs perform at the level of a second-year resident), their own personal expectations for ideal performance in the clinical arena, and the expectations of those to whom they report in the work setting:

I just assumed she [the NP] knew everything. . . . If she said something, it was gospel. . . . It was the way she carried herself — she just had a presence about her. . . . And I remember when I started and she'd go through the list — GSW, GSW, GSW — and I'm like, "Oh my word. This is like ER. I can never do this". . . . There wasn't even a resident affiliated with the team; she was the resident and the nurse. I didn't even see the nursing part of what she did; I just knew she was a nurse who knew — God — more than I'd ever know, and seemed as knowledgeable as a physician and worked in a field that boggles my mind, but she was able to pull it all together. And it wasn't until long afterwards that I could see her doing the nursing piece, the counselling with the patients and their families because I was just too caught up in the medical efficiency piece she did. . . . I didn't even know that I didn't see it that way until I'd been in the NP role for quite a while.

NPs experience an acute awareness of how others may see them. There is a sense of split between the "I" who experiences the world through their own eyes and the "me" whom they see through the eyes of others. As they squirm under the Other's gaze, they fear being "found out" for who they "really" are behind their façade. They are afraid that if others were to know the truth about them, those Others would feel betrayed or disappointed, with the consequence that they could be rejected or disgraced. They tend to live with a sense of dread and foreboding that it will only be a matter of time before they are found out. The result is often a sense of incredulity that others actually have placed their confidence in them:

> And I always thought it was strange that when I would see a patient and would say to the patient, "Do you want to see the [medical specialist] today?" and they would say, "No, I don't want to see him today". . . . And the physicians would seem quite confident for that to happen, that I would have my list of patients to see, the resident had theirs and the physicians had theirs. . . . And it always felt so strange that they seemed to have an overwhelming confidence in me. They probably had more confidence in my decisions than I did at the time. I always felt strange about that.

But perhaps being an impostor goes even deeper. NPs may feel that there is a layer surrounding and concealing their real identity when they can only focus on what they are learning and doing within the medical sphere of their role. At some level, NPs are aware that although they are playing a role, they do not yet embody it. It may be that they do not yet completely identify with it. In this sense they are "betwixt and between."

The more we identify with a role, the less separate and distinct we feel from it. Conversely, the less we identify with a role, the more aware we become that we are not the role we play. Possibly, feeling like an impostor means that NPs are not yet able to identify with what they are doing because it doesn't yet feel morally like who they are. This might cause them to feel even more distanced from their nursing colleagues. It has been recognized that instrumental work and rational thinking stand outside the philosophical foundations of nursing when they are not embedded in a relational ethic of care. Wicks (1998) wrote that nursing celebrates closeness and connectedness in a relational approach to care that links the physical with the emotional aspects of caring. Perhaps NPs become uncomfortable when they experience a disconnection of themselves and their role — the experience of being lost.

The irony about being betwixt and between is that many NPs make interesting discoveries about themselves as nurses during this period. Being lost is a form of un-knowing what was previously known and knowing things anew, a constant trying on of roles for size, of evaluating how well they fit. As Altrows (2002, p. 9) explained, "When we find a role that suits us, we may become so identified with the role and so accustomed to it that we forget that it is a role at all. It is as if we become asleep to our true selves." Perhaps NPs feel like impostors as they become aware of the ever-shifting tension between themselves and the roles that they play. Without this awareness, they risk losing themselves in the role, thereby losing the freedom to try on new roles and discard those that no longer fit. "In the end, our experience of feeling like an impostor may awaken us to our true selves and what it means to be free" (Altrows, 2002, p. 9).

NPs recognize what it means to be a nurse through what they do, by having it brought to their attention by physicians, and by what they miss, such as being connected and being a provider of holistic care. This recognition puts them on alert. As if they were standing in front of a mirror, they notice many things about themselves that they did not see before. A recognition of "me" occurs. Yet this "me" is not the "self" they are familiar with; the "mirror" that they are facing is a distorting mirror, and the person in front of them is not who they had expected to see. Some NPs may even become cautious and carefully adjust themselves to create a better image depending on the community of practice with which they are engaged. This is not an easy period. Feeling like strangers, they cannot satisfy themselves with what they do. Their eyes become so keen that all they can see is their flaws and who they are not. Not only are they strangers to others, but they are also becoming strangers to themselves. They are lost. They wonder who they should be.

NPs come to their role understanding their way of being in the health care world from a nursing perspective, an understanding built on a tradition of holism, a perspective more often particularistic and subjective rather than objective and distant, as is the medical perspective. But under the circumstance of becoming an NP, a person's focus shifts from dwelling within the healing model, with its emphasis on knowing the patient fully and optimizing health and comfort, to the notion of patient as body to be observed, known, and treated, using the language of domination and control, as is evident in the scientific model of medicine (Gadow, 1980). NPs spend their days focused on deductive reasoning, constructing hypotheses, and using established procedures and algorithms. During this initial period, the dominant aspects of their role are both mechanistic and reductionistic. They are continuously informed that if they have the right facts and a full understanding of pathophysiologic processes, they will be able to predict and control events. They are explicitly told to "stop thinking like a nurse" by their physician colleagues. Through their concentration on increasingly detailed aspects of physical dysfunction, it is not only easy for them to lose sight of the patient as specific individual, it is almost essential that this happens. In this way, their focus is kept clear and their energy is consolidated while they learn what they need in order to perform safely when clinically caring for their patients.

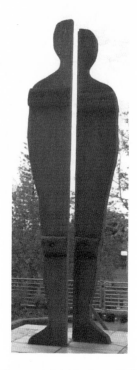

FIG. 2. Sculpture of Split Person, Adelaide, Australia (Photo: J. Rashotte, 2005).

But this language and focus for being, however necessary, often feels foreign and wrong. It involves a detachment or disconnection from the patients' suffering and pain, and they struggle with it, even though "the art of describing facts is the supreme art in medicine: everything pales before it" (Foucault, 1994, p. 146). Some NPs are torn between their admiration for the "coolness and presence of mind" needed to perform well in this role, particularly under pressure, and a fear that to acquire that level of knowledge and skill will require the sacrifice of the philosophical tenets of nursing. In order to master the knowledge domains within medicine, along with being situated within the medical world, albeit on the edges, they wonder if they will have to give up their connections to nurses, nursing, patients, and patients' families. It seems to contradict one of the main goals of the journey — to be more connected to the Other. While in medicine involvement is a by-product of the quest for knowledge, in nursing it is a central and pleasurable part of the work (Wicks, 1998). In this sense, whole days, weeks, and months spent predominantly in discourses that focus only on objectification of the patient, with limited time for relational activities, is in opposition to what NPs traditionally value and thereby creates an internal struggle or tension. Are they co-opting their values related to nursing for goals that are not achievable except at the expense of those values? What do they have to lose in order to gain?

Inner conflict may lead to great distress. In fact, learning to care for patients from a medical perspective is not only destabilizing, but it is also polarizing. NPs experience this struggle as needing to make a choice between a practice incorporating autonomy and skill that is based on the scientific paradigm and a practice within a "cosmology of healing" (Wicks, 1998, p. 72). Being lost is experienced as a dichotomy of two mutually exclusive and contradictory paths. From this new viewpoint, their past is severed and they have become two unconnected pieces. Thinking like a physician is experienced as oppositional to thinking like a nurse. It is experienced as moving to the physician side of health care, which implies necessarily leaving the nursing side. Am I a nurse or am I a physician replacement?

Being lost makes NPs feel like their own "self" is falling away, and their old self clashes with their newly discovered self. As noted previously, there are two Is, perceived as dichotomous, bipolar, and opposing each other. There is the nursing "I," with whom they are familiar and feel connected, the "I" they enjoyed and were proud of and wished to promote and enhance when they chose to depart on the journey to becoming an NP, and they do not want to let it go. The other "I," the "I" engaged in traditional medical acts and seen externally, is a stranger, like a distorted figure who always reappears during moments of disconnection. They feel they cannot accept this "stranger" self because they do not want it, but they cannot reject it because it is becoming part of their new self — the new knowledge and skills that they are acquiring are necessary to being more challenged, more visible, and more in control. Being lost means NPs possess a disorganized inner world and inhabit an unconnected outer world, and as a result much of their world as an NP is experienced as paradoxical.

To be a castaway is to be a point perpetually at the centre of a circle. However much things may appear to change — the sea may shift from whisper to rage, the sky might go from fresh blue to blinding white to darkest black — the geometry never changes. Your gaze is always a radius. The circumference is ever great. In fact, the circles multiply. To be a castaway is to be caught in a harrowing ballet of circles. You are at the centre of one circle, while above you two opposing circles spin about. The sun distresses you like a crowd, a noisy, invasive crowd that makes you cup your ears, that makes you close your eyes, that makes you want to hide. The moon distresses you by silently reminding you of your solitude; you open your eyes wide to escape your loneliness. When you look up, you sometimes wonder if at the centre of a solar storm, if in the middle of the Sea of Tranquillity, there isn't another one like you also looking up, also trapped by geometry, also struggling with fear, rage, madness, hopelessness, apathy. (Martel, 2002, p. 239)

Operating from a dichotomous position is not dissimilar to this passage in Yann Martel's (2002) critically acclaimed contemporary novel *The Life of Pi*. The story concerns the transformational journey of a sixteen-year old boy named Pi Patel, who, after the sinking of a cargo ship, finds himself alone for many months on the only surviving lifeboat, with a group of wild animals. Being a castaway, as Pi is, offers an example of being "caught up in grim and exhausting opposites" (Martel, 2002, p. 240). On the one hand, what NPs originally seek on their journey seems to have collapsed into pieces and becomes elusive to grasp. On the other hand, this new world is experienced as gigantic and overwhelming, making them feel small and dwarfed in the unknown but powerful world of medicine. How can NPs feel that they have no centre when they also feel as if they are perpetually at the centre of the circle?

> And I started writing orders and people started doing them, which I found very odd. Why are they doing what I'm telling them to do? Don't they know I'm just like them? Here I'm in this role, I felt very much — not powerful, but you know that you have the final say, and what you say goes, and people are actually listening to you.

When NPs begin to experience the overwhelming nature of carrying the responsibility that comes with autonomy of practice, they immediately seek solace in the ultimate responsibility belonging to the staff physician. When they are called upon to defend their choice of action, the visibility is frightening. But surprisingly they can also feel moments of exhilaration.

> When you're first doing [intubations] you're not sure that you can repeat it even though you've done the skills; like can you do it under this pressure and can you do it in that situation? But at the same time, when you did it, it was like, "Oh, I did it! I accomplished it! It's great! This is such a great day, I did this and this."

NPs feel excited and exhilarated with their success in the advanced instrumental nature of their practice, and they feel that they have made a difference in the lives of their patients. It is during these fleeting moments that they experience real pleasure, a glimmer of the perfect fit for which they are searching, a feeling of being close to home. Is this swing of the pendulum from exhilaration to terror not the worst pair of opposites with which to live, particularly when they are experienced in the same moment? For indeed these two opposites do not remain distinct. Life at the time of being lost is not much of a life. Pi reflects, "It is like an end game in chess, a game with few pieces. The elements couldn't be more simple, nor the stakes higher. Physically it is extraordinarily arduous, and morally it is killing. . . . You reach a point where you're at the bottom of hell, yet you have your arms crossed and a smile on your face, and you feel you're the luckiest person on earth" (Martel, 2002, p. 241).

In this time of being lost, NPs undergo a disintegration, and a reshaping of self is needed to regain peace and confidence. In so doing, they undergo a profound and irreversible change. The process is threatening because they have to alter their identities in order to accept this transformation.

Staying Afloat

During this time of tension and struggle, NPs are being called to inhabit the present by seizing the opportunity to listen to their consciences and to take responsibility for making something of themselves on the basis of who they already are (Heidegger, 1962, pp. 318, 344). This may mean choosing a very different course for their nursing career or struggling to stay afloat. In either case, they must gain a clearer understanding of who they are, what is truly important to them, and what they need to do in the nursing world. They must enter into "the situation" (Heidegger, 1962,

p. 346) to find an authentic way of being. As Heidegger argued, genuine decisions involve taking a risk in the context of a unique situation. During this time, NPs are being continuously requested to authentically reaffirm their desire to be NPs. If they choose to struggle to stay afloat, they are ultimately called into action.

The turbulence experienced in being adrift creates a need for stability that is achieved through the influence of positive forces. NPs use what Heitz, Steiner, and Burman, (2004) referred to as "optimistic self-talk"— comments such as *You've got to keep working* and *You're prepared to do this* — a form of internal reinforcement, a personal coping mechanism, that helps them maintain a positive mental attitude.

Despite the turbulence encountered, staying afloat becomes a self-reinforcing motivator. The will to succeed is a matter of pride for NPs, a need to hold on to the belief in their abilities and the right to discover the sense of fulfilment for which they are searching. Staying afloat is about refusing to be a pawn in the health care game of resource management. Preparing the way for others to follow and being successful in meeting this challenge are some of the rewards of journeying through being adrift, and NPs hold fast to the possibility of such attainment. Living through the struggles and tensions is perceived as a necessary sacrifice in order to experience the rewards: "I think the challenge of being the first graduate nurse practitioner in the province was something that keeps you going. You say, 'Well, we're going to be the first ones out; we're going to be out of the gate before everybody else.' Also, I think it's a bit of a pride thing to keep going. Plus you always think that it's going to get better with time."

All of the feelings associated with being uncertain need to be quickly contained if the NP is to survive the experience of being adrift. NPs must actively employ ways and means to successfully face and overcome their uncertainties. Therefore, if being uncertain is seen as a challenge, then there is a requirement to engage in a battle to subdue it: "I guess the challenge is what keeps me going. I'm one of those 'keep-going' persons. . . . If I find that the challenge is becoming uncomfortable then maybe I need to do something about it."

Jumping into the fray, studying and using their desire to promote learning and professional growth become strategies for coping with their worries. Perhaps they feel as Melville (1992, p. 25) wrote in *Moby Dick*: "I have swum through oceans and sailed through libraries." NPs speak about the need to simply immerse themselves in a constant state of learning; as such, academic learning is seen as a positive force. They recognize that the theoretical knowledge and skill that they have acquired in the classroom setting is but the tip of the iceberg. In fact, one NP said, "the more you learn, the more you want to learn. Oh, I wish I knew a bit more and then a bit more, and then a bit more after that. So I did a lot of reading."

But the key issue during this time is to be able to mobilize problem-solving skills enough to function and to meet the responsibilities of diagnosing and treating patients. Doing and learning become essential partners. NPs recognize that theoretical knowledge, or "knowing that," must be translated into "knowing how" (Schön, 1987), and immersion in their work as clinical practitioners is critical: "I think sometimes you just have to pluck up the courage to just say it, just write it. . . . I mean, my pockets are full of stuff because I always want to have a back-up if I'm not sure. I never write stuff if I'm not sure about it . . . so I have the NP's *Guide to Diagnosis and Treatment* or whatever and my Palm Pilot."

NPs strive to create a safety net or lifeline that will protect both self and others; it is a way to deal with their fear of harming their patients through their possible mistakes in clinical decision-making. This safety net comes in a variety of forms, most of which are used repeatedly, frequently, and concurrently. Checking and rechecking their work and asking the same question multiple times or of multiple people are natural responses to being worried, and they encourage confirmation that the right action will be taken. There is a hope that someone will be alert to a potential error and will catch them before they do harm: "I came back; I reviewed the chart; I looked over everything and decided that yes it is done right. This is what should be done; everything is correct; okay, now stop it; now go home. But you know, there's one or two things that just pop into my head and it is like, well it's either go back or I'm up all night reading a CPS. . . . Sometimes that's what I have to do."

Even engaging in the diagnostic reasoning process comes to be understood as part of the safety net. Examining all possible causes for the patient's signs and symptoms becomes the way to ensure no stone has gone unturned: "Your assessment might lead you to believe this is what the issue is, but you always want to build a safety net in case you make a mistake. . . . The focus is always on protecting the patient and making sure that the patient is not exposed to unnecessary risk."

For the first few years, the NPs' priority is to get the knowledge and skill that they need to perform safely. Weeks into the new role, they begin to develop their own navigational charts. Being practical people, trained and experienced in the ways of nursing, many NPs look toward immediate development of policies and procedures in the form of protocols, clinical guidelines, or medical directives that serve as maps to help them safely navigate through the clinical decision-making process that is required of them:

And I developed protocols for certain things that I do that would sort of guide me along. Like, how I deal with somebody who's bleeding, or how would I deal with somebody who is having arrhythmias, and what pathway would you take, and having the clinical guidelines with the knowledge and the theory behind what you do, and those kind of things. Versus just doing what the doctor tells me I should do, or this is what the doctor does so this is what I should do.

These guidelines and directives serve to anchor NPs to something that feels stable and sure at a time when they feel as if they are drifting. If artifacts and practices are not available for adoption — which normally enables engagement with our community of practice and contributes to shape the relations of accountability by which we define our actions as *competent* (Wenger, 1998) — then they must be constructed through a process of negotiation. The interesting outcome of the formalization of these new practices is that the process allows NPs to engage with others around the dimensions of the various practices in which they may be involved. This then affords them the power to negotiate their enterprises and thus shape the context in which they will work, and they begin to experience an identity of competence. In addition, the creative imagination required to construct the guidelines and directives is anchored in social interactions and communal experiences and thus fosters a mode of belonging.

The following example demonstrates the construction of these artifacts. Within the first month of being in the role of NP, "June" was informed by her director of nursing that the hospital could not legally support her in any expanded role activities. Attempting to deal with the mixed message of "do the job but don't step outside the scope" was clearly a challenge of being a pioneer. However, this challenge set in motion the creative process of negotiating a scope of practice that would be acceptable with respect to both her subspecialty and broader institutional communities of practice, as well as establishing a structure that would legally protect both her and the institution. Creating such a context in which to proceed with her working life while maintaining a sense of self that she could live with in this new role shows how NPs develop a sense of belonging and their sense of identity in larger contexts — historical, social, cultural, and institutional — with specific resources and constraints:

One of the things that became clear very quickly was that in order to be effective I needed to have medical directives. They'd never been devised at the hospital before. . . . There wasn't a lot written on them at that time. . . . And I said, 'Okay. Well we need to do this because I have to have some structure to order analgesics, to order IV fluid. I can't just be ordering these things. There has to be a structure that protects me legally, protects the institution legally.' And because there was no template at that time, although I did receive advice from the College of Nurses, I developed what seemed workable for me which was approved by the physicians.

June's story also illustrates that where there are obstacles there is an Athena ready to assist NPs in navigating them. Sometimes NPs have to actively seek such assistance, while at other times they need only to seize the opportunities that are presented, a finding revealed in the work by Reay, Golden-Biddle, and GermAnn (2006). As June further shared:

But [the medical directive] was blocked by my director at the time because she wasn't too sure about it because, while she'd acknowledged that I needed it, she wasn't sure if it was the right time to present it to the organization. So I got quite frustrated because I was practising and I was trying to find a way to make sure that I was covered legally. . . . So what I actually had to do was to run around using the political structure. I actually had made good friends with a nurse who was on the committee . . . that looked at all practice-related stuff . . . and she said, "Why don't we just do a back-door thing. You give it to me and I'll take it to the committee for approval without going through the director. . . . Once it's approved, she can't say anything". . . . I was quite happy when that got approved and then I could sort of be on firmer footing to do some of these things.

June noted, "When you're the first one there, there's no process, and people don't really know what the process should be," but as a result of meeting this pioneering challenge, policies, procedures, and protocols were now put in place for others to use. There was also the beginning of a shared history, one that facilitates new NPs' sense of belonging within this institution's community of practice.

NPs, like "Cody", who work in a province where the concept of medical directives is non-existent, and where legislation denies them the right to advance their scope of practice independently into the arena of prescriptive and diagnostic authority, describe how they "need to constantly cover" themselves, all the while feeling like they are "walking on eggs." Not being covered or fully certified, they feel they're in between two groups, constantly confused as to their status and frustrated that they have not been recognized as an entity.

> Giving a diagnosis is a big No in our province. But how can you decide on a lab test, how can you decide a plan of treatment if you can't say that you saw pneumonia on the X-ray? . . . So we say it's a pneumonia not yet diagnosed. . . . Then, actually, I have to go to one of the fellows and say maybe we need to start antibiotics because the child has a fever, because the white count is high, because of the type of secretions, and because of the findings on the X-ray. And then I write the order and I have to get the fellow or the staff physician to countersign it.

Because NPs like Cody do not have a solid basis in terms of legal recognition or the use of medical directives, they create a safety line by "always backing themselves up" by having everything countersigned. But as a consequence, they frequently find themselves struggling with the tension of "playing politics and doing footwork" for the physicians, both of which negate the raison d'être of the journey.

I cannot work without my physician colleagues being there. Within this hospital we only work as an NP when there's an attending physician in-house. So this makes it a relationship where I totally depend on them to be here and in a sense they depend on me because a lot of what I do is footwork — call for tests, call consultants, speak to people. And sometimes that's frustrating. It just depends on how I look at it. It depends if it's a priority for me. If I see it as this is my patient, this is the plan of care, this is where I want to go, then it doesn't bother me because that's what I do. If I'm calling people and doing things which I don't think are necessary for my patient or appropriate, then I feel like I'm doing footwork. . . . I guess the footwork is when I'm told, "You will call so and so and say such and such a thing." "Well, pick up the phone and do it yourself". . . . I feel like a secretary. . . . And it doesn't challenge me to move beyond or that I'm in a relationship where I feel that what I have to say or what I have to offer is important or valued.

NPs argue that the strongest determinant of whether they are going to be successful is the physicians they are going to work with. One NP declared, "Those acute-care NPs who have been assigned to work with lousy physicians with bad attitudes are struggling before they even set foot in the door." NPs who are "left out there just hanging in the wind to make diagnoses and clinical decisions on their own, be they right or wrong," often come to see themselves as working for their physician rather than with them, as "physician extenders." Unfortunately, in these circumstances some NPs are unable to stay afloat. Some experience depression, which results in the need to take a leave of absence early on in the process. Therefore establishing open dialogue and a rapport with the staff physicians in their practice as quickly as possible is essential to their well-being. Being aligned with staff physicians is one means by which they create a lifeline, and they work hard to develop and maintain this alignment. Alignment helps them to manage the level of complexity in their clinical practice that they do not yet know how to manage and gives them a sense of hope that they can stay afloat.

The lifeline emerges from belief that the physician will always be there, recognizing their limitations, helping them to navigate through all the trials and tribulations of clinical management of the patient. This is experienced as a feeling that they will never really be on their own, a sense of the physician being present to provide reassurance, or a sense of security that they will do the right thing and that they are providing the best standard of care. Physician presence as a lifeline, either through being there physically or being with them by making room for dialogue, conveys to the NPs that they have not been abandoned, particularly during this time of being disconnected. In the face of uncertainty and the subsequent state of worry that emerges, NPs must turn to the outside to make that which is in doubt certain, or at least less uncertain.

Physicians' willingness to share information, teach, coach, and demonstrate what needs to be done implies a desire to nurture the NPs' professional growth and development in the direct clinical practice dimension of the NPs' role. Lacking confidence in their abilities to clinically care for patients, NPs need their fears and concerns dispelled in almost every new situation by having their opinions and impressions confirmed as correct. Although they realize that they must eventually make decisions independently, the lifeline seems most secure when they believe that they will not be penalized if they cannot make a decision. They feel instead that they can "check in" or "run something by" their staff physicians any time they have questions or concerns. Physician presence creates a trusting relationship that prevents NPs' fears and worries from becoming paralyzing, thus allowing them to test their abilities and eventually to risk carrying the responsibility they seek:

> When you're first doing the role and carrying the responsibility, you need to have a system in place for support. You need to have physicians who don't mind you popping in, maybe even several times a day, to say, "I just want to run this by you; what do you think about this? Is that right?" And they'll confirm it or they'll say, "Yeah, that's right 90 percent of the time except in this case". . . . Or I'll go back and say, "What do you think I could've done differently?" One of the physicians is very good at that, very supportive. . . . I remember, I went to him once and I said, "I don't know what else to do. This is the problem. I've done this. I've done this. I've done this. I did this and it's still not fixed. What else can I do?" And he looked at me and he said, "Witchcraft. [laughs] Like there's nothing else that you could've done." So just that reinforcement from him that no, there's nothing else here to the situation.

The length and tautness of the lifeline is always determined by negotiation in the NP–physician relationship. While some NPs have the expectation that the physician will supervise them until the NP expresses comfort with managing the situation, others desire the freedom to take risks without the physician standing over them. But in either case, they are grateful and feel fortunate when their physician colleagues understand what they need, are there to support them as necessary, and then are willing to let them become independent through a gradual weaning process, all the while being willing to be available whenever their assistance is required.

> This bi-weekly meeting with my consultants is something that I've created to get my questions answered, and if it's urgent then there's a resident on call, or I'll even call my staff consultant. You always have the lifeline of the phone. . . . And just being clear, as all nurses have to be, that either I just want to chat with them to get their reassurance and they can stay at their desk, or "No you need to come and see this patient."

There is a clear understanding and appreciation that the lifeline available to acute-care NPs is different from that available to NPs working in primary care. Some NPs feel more protected in the hospital because if they are unsure, they always have someone to call. Noting that their patient populations can "be so wide with diseases that are seen only once in awhile," or rare conditions that are not straightforward, some NPs admit that they would feel uncomfortable with full autonomy. Because the Canadian Public Hospitals Act provides that the final authority lies with the admitting physician, there is a sense of security in the knowledge that NPs do not bear the ultimate responsibility and authority for the clinical management of the patient. Yet, tension arises as a result of their living with the paradox of searching for independence and more control while holding on to the comfort of the security of the physician's presence.

> I think I feel more protected in the hospital because, if I ever am not sure, I've got somebody to call. I mean even if there's not always a resident, there's always a fellow or a surgeon that I can double-check with. . . . So if I were working out in the community or way up North and you're the only one there, it's either sink or swim. But I think that would be a really valuable experience too. I'd love to go to the North, to be there for three months just to know that it's me, me, and me. . . . So I'd say the fear is less when you work in the hospital because you're not alone. You're working in a team. However, you don't have the ultimate authority to make decisions like the physicians do.

Unfortunately, staying afloat becomes more of a struggle when NPs do not trust the staff physicians with whom they are partnered. Doubtful that the physician will back them up if a mistake is made, they contain their scope of practice to what they feel they can manage without any risk, frequently defaulting to the physician. In these situations, the strength of the lifeline — its ability to enable NPs to engage in their work and learn to take the risks necessary to become more independent — is also its danger. The lifeline becomes a cord that ties them to the medical team in a dependent and disabling manner when fear of loss of their approval and the need for their affirmation becomes more important than the goals for which they strive.

Creating a lifeline through an alignment with their physician colleagues not only expands the scope of NPs' influence on their world within nursing, but also gives them new and different understandings about those with whom they now engage in some shared activities. Along with feeling privileged to develop a personal relationship with staff physicians, to "really know each other better," NPs also undergo a growing awareness of and appreciation for some of the experiences that residents live through on their journeys to becoming independent medical practitioners.

> I think a lot of residents are scared. Some of them will voice it
> right out but not many because it's not very doctor-like. . . .
> I think that's one way that I'm privileged. I think a lot of them
> when you see them on the unit wouldn't appear that way. But some
> of the residents, they'll be asking me, "Do you think I did this
> right? Do you think that's right? Do you think that's correct?"
> And I think that's because they understand how scary it is.

As a result, NPs begin to rethink their own experiences and way of engaging in and contributing to the practices of their communities as an NP. Perhaps because of this growing understanding they do not feel quite as isolated; rather, they sense a connectedness with others who struggle as they do, others who are also attempting to survive in their quest for a career, albeit a different one. In spite of the curriculum, discipline, and exhortation, the learning that is most personally transformative for NPs turns out to be that which involves membership in these various communities of practice, in which there is a sense of shared lived experience that can amplify their sense of the possible. Because they are able to consider a new mode of belonging to this community of practice, new ways of seeing themselves as NPs open up that may ultimately reconstruct their experiences of power and identity.

NPs quickly learn that the lifeline becomes even stronger through the creation of team solidarity. Drawing on their nursing foundations, they turn toward the belief that clinical decisions need to be "spread out over a number of people" through the formation of partnerships, rather than being made in isolation. Nurses, physicians, social workers, physiotherapists, dieticians, pharmacists, respiratory therapists, and others, including the patient and family, are seen as friends whose input must be taken into account in the decision-making process. When this is done, there is a sense of relief that treatment plans are "on the right track" and possible mistakes will be foreseen by others before they are made.

> I often rely on my nursing colleagues. . . . I ordered magnesium not so long ago. Magnesium is not something we give very often here, so I ordered it with the protocol, and then I went to the nurse and said, "Well look, this is what I'm ordering for this patient; I used this protocol; Is this the way you understand it? Does this order make sense to you?". . . So I think that's one way that I can help myself not be constantly worried. So I think my nursing colleague is a good safeguard for me.

Striving together becomes an important enterprise (Wenger, 1998), not only as a mechanism for preventing mistakes, but also as part of NPs' larger quest for a viable identity. They must find ways to organize their lives with their immediate colleagues and patients in order to learn what they need to do. Thus they develop or preserve a sense of themselves that they can live with and so have some inkling of belonging, all the while learning to fulfill the requirements of their employers and patients. For example, they quickly find that they need to cultivate respect with nurses by being effective and efficient from day one, even though they lack the requisite knowledge and skill to be able to do this in their new role. Thus, they strive to create opportunities to make and maintain connections with their nursing colleagues, stressing the importance of earning their respect, which takes a great deal of time and effort. Some do so by attending nursing handover rounds, appreciating that the areas of concern for nursing are of significance to the plan of care, as well as the fact that nurses usually have greater depth of information about their patients than the residents. In addition, they enjoy the camaraderie that takes place during this event. Other NPs make conscious efforts to be part of the nursing team by negotiating the time that will work best for them to undertake the procedures required by patients. Some ensure that they remain involved in traditional nursing activities, such as suctioning patients' secretions, emptying bedpans, and reprogramming intravenous pumps as the need arises, demonstrating that they want to work side by side with nurses, not above them, just as they wish to work side by side with the physician, not below them. Some NPs invite nurses to participate in writing orders by creating opportunities for their input, thus ensuring that their concerns are heard, and respect for their ideas is demonstrated in a way that empowers them, so the safety net is strengthened and the relationship with nurses is solidified in a new type of partnership.

It's not easy to flip over to writing on the physician's order sheets and then directing your colleagues in terms of giving them orders as well. . . . But you develop techniques of how to get around that. Yes, there's specific directions from a litigation and liability perspective that need to be written on the physician order sheet, and most of those directives are medical directives, but others of them are inviting the nurse to be part of the decision making and order writing as, well, not just being a scribe. . . . So, in terms of inviting the nurse — "Well, what do you think of the plan? We've had this team discussion so let's summarize and I'll write these orders on the physician order sheet. So NPO, the IV solution, the TFI. How does this look to you? We've calculated out that the TFI's going to be about 8 ml per kilo per hour. What does that mean to you?" And having them check them — "Does this look okay to you? Is this what we talked about?". . . And I'm not telling the nurse what to do. I mean these are medical orders, but we have to work together and they've had their input on how they are going to look; I'm just putting them down in black and white.

Despite living in a potentially turbulent time during which they experience being disconnected from that which is familiar and feels like home, NPs find that the work of staying afloat allows them to also experience moments of undeniable joy and satisfaction, moments — however fleeting — of awe and wonder at the things that they do and accomplish. It is these moments that provide them with a glimpse of what the future holds, the possibility of finding the perfect fit somewhere on the horizon.

Polaris, my guide
Shining on the thorny path
Painfully traversed

— Mika Yoshimoto (2008, p. 23)

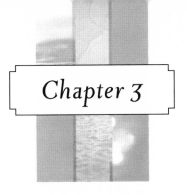

Chapter 3

Being a Nurse Practitioner

"I'm not afraid of storms, for I'm learning how to sail my ship."
— Amy, in *Little Women* by Louisa May Alcott

The first time I felt like a real nurse practitioner was my first night
solo with a real critically ill infant and getting through all of the
trials and tribulations and then thinking that I had made it through
the night. It was a baby that the transport team had brought in
from a local hospital. . . . We suspected that this infant could be
in overwhelming strep sepsis and was deteriorating rapidly. . . .
At the beginning it was mostly the skills . . . so I worked with the
respiratory therapist, the attending physician, and two of the nurses
who were going to be the admission nurses and we had everything
ready. I had all the orders done, we had all our calculations, we had
all our pumps all lined up and labelled and so it was going to be as
efficient an admission as we could possibly have or that we could
have control over. . . . So then getting the airway efficiently, getting

the lines in and pushing fluids, and getting the orders, and managing a cardiac arrest, those kinds of critical things, the technical part of it, and the sense of accomplishment with having that expertise of being able to do those skills. . . . So being able to be successful, being able to facilitate such a critically ill infant through admission and stabilization and the family as well. I mean, it's tough being able to do that with the parents in the room. . . . I don't think you ever get really comfortable with it, but the fact is, they need to be there. So it's having their trust and their confidence in that you are doing your best that you can for their baby. Then to have the attending physician's confidence that I could manage this type of patient competently also was a professional compliment I guess. . . . But it was a team effort. . . . It was a real sense of togetherness. . . . There was a real sense of success and accomplishment and that we made a difference in this family's and this baby's lives. And I think that had to be one of the most rewarding parts, knowing I was a key player in that team dynamic. It was an incredible feeling.

Through time, experience, and reflective engagement, NPs gradually journey through being adrift to fully being an acute-care NP. "Feeling like an NP" occurs as a result of being able to do direct clinical practice, which is experienced as being competent, confident, comfortable, committed, connected, and content. The above quotation demonstrates how becoming an NP is a complex process that combines doing, talking, thinking, feeling, and belonging to a clinical practice team that recognizes, acknowledges, and values designated nurses who perform clinical components of practice traditionally carried out by physicians.

Gradually, NPs gain new knowledge and skills in clinically managing patients. This occurs with the help of, and despite any hindrance from, members in their work communities. Opportunities to care for patients with similar health problems facilitate the solidification and refinement of previously learned knowledge. NPs commonly journey two or three years, sometimes even longer, with an intense focus in the same clinical specialty, encountering the same types of practice issues, and working with the same medical and nursing team, before they feel confident, competent, and comfortable in direct clinical practice. The time may be less for those who have advanced clinical skills or bear increased responsibility prior to becoming NPs, such as neonatal transport nurses or CNSs working in the same specialty service with the same team.

Being competent, confident, and comfortable — feelings that are so integral to each other that it is often almost impossible to distinguish between them — are the performance markers that must be recognized by oneself as well as others before NPs can successfully journey through being adrift. These feelings enable NPs to be committed and connected to their patients, patients' families, and members of their community of practice in a way that is morally acceptable to the NP. NPs can now experience being content. These feelings, combined with a sense of belonging, of discovering more, and of being able to make a difference begin to prevail and, as a result, they identify themselves as being NPs. Some even find the perfect fit at this point in their journey.

As a result of experiencing clinical practice in this new way, NPs are able to shift their perspective away from the internal polarized discourse and struggle (*Am I a physician replacement or a nurse or neither?*) toward an acknowledgement that harmony may exist within previously perceived opposites and a new identity may arise from previously antagonistic patterns of practice. As a result of experiencing practice in this new way, each NP is able to experience a coherent sense of self. Drawing on the thinking of philosopher Charles Taylor (1991a, pp. 305–306), we can view this time as the period during which NPs shift away from questioning who they are (because they do not know how to react when it comes to questions of values and issues of importance for them as nurses) toward situating themselves in ethical space, where they are able to measure up to their obligations. Of ultimate relevance, they are able to meet these obligations in such a way that they now cultivate self-descriptions that include moral or ethical self-characterizations of what is truly important to them. This does not imply that tensions, conflicts, or concessions no longer exist. Rather, NPs now begin to acknowledge that the knowledge and skills that they have acquired from both medical and nursing models of care ultimately enhance their practice. Consequently, they gradually experience a transformation in their lived identity — an identity that continues to be shaped by recognition and that is crucially dependent on dialogical relations with others, for as Taylor (1994) reminds us, "There is no such thing as inward generation [of identity], monologically understood. . . . We define our identity always in dialogue with, sometimes in struggle against, the things our significant others want to see in us" (pp. 32–33).

Being Competent

Competence, a word derived from the Latin word competere (com meaning "together with" and petere meaning to "aim at") is defined as having a sufficient or adequate degree of knowledge and skill to do a task effectively and safely. Being competent necessarily moves NPs beyond taking on the title to the realm of doing what NPs do, to forming a community of practice that permits mutual engagement in the work that needs to be accomplished, and entertaining certain relations with other communities of practice. In this process, they find a personal meaning in the title "NP." As Wenger (1998, p. 152) observed, when we handle ourselves competently, experience competence, and are recognized as competent, we begin to feel that we are full members of the community of practice in which we are engaged. These dimensions of competence then become dimensions of our identity. In this sense, identity is an experience and a display of competence. Consequently, knowledge and skill must be transformed into action; knowing must become doing, which is what Benner, Hooper-Kyriakidis, and Stannard (1999) and Schön (1983, 1987) referred to as the act of transforming "knowing that" into 'knowing how," or the acquisition of knowing-in-action. Specifically, NPs need to be considered by themselves and others to be fit or suitably and sufficiently qualified to independently carry out the task of medically managing the patients within their specialty of practice. This occurs through a process of affirmation during which NPs prove they have passed initiation into the traditions of the medical community of practitioners and the practice world that they inhabit by demonstrating what Schön (1987) described as "the community's conventions, constraints, language, and appreciative systems, their repertoire of exemplars, systematic knowledge, and patterns of knowing-in-action." (p. 36)

In the more accurate sense of the meaning of the word *competere*, NPs, physicians, nurses, and even patients strive together to bring NPs to their rightful place within their larger communities of practice. Being competent must be formed within a context of mutual engagement; it is an outcome of a joint enterprise in which there is a shared or mutually negotiated range of expectations for performance. Being engaged in action with other people in the performance of clinical care activities means that all members of the community must come to some understanding about what being a competent NP means, even if this understanding is not articulated. Community members must not only recognize but also acknowledge competence in the NPs' performances. NPs must then experience themselves as competent, as observed in others' recognition of them combined with an appreciation of others' performances of similar activities and as compared to their own observations of their performance. Undeniably, the unspoken, taken-for-granted sense of what competence looks like from the Other's point of view quickly seeps into their expectations:

Well from the nurses' point of view, I mean you're expected to be competent in the skills that they want you to do. You should be able to get IVS when nobody else can. So you do these procedures with the expectation that you're going to get them and that you'll be competent in the extra skills, and that they can go to you for a decision and get a decision.

What does NP clinical competence look like in action? How is competence affirmed? How do NPs experience competence? How does it relate to being confident and comfortable?

Being competent is initiated with the endowment of both the legal authority and the qualifications to grant admissibility into the medical sphere. Graduation from a legitimately recognized education program authorizes NPs, administrators of employing institutions, and physicians with whom they are partnered to publicly claim that NPs hold an officially recognized position and are qualified by their convincing demonstrations of special attributes, skills, and knowledge to intercede in the matters of disease and death, a position traditionally held by physicians alone. Licensed status adds a further recognition of competence by investing an official social status through a symbol of bureaucratic enterprise. These official sanctions bring about a "professed authority" that demands that practitioners "project an image of trustworthy competence to their clients" (Haas and Shaffir, 1987, p. 1).

Yet, attaining certification or NP licensure does not automatically result in NPs being able to handle themselves competently. Competence develops only with experience and the recognition that theoretical knowledge has been translated into an acceptable form of action. Well-known motivational speaker Dale Carnegie (1964) wrote that there are four ways in which we have contact with the world and are classified and evaluated by others: what we do, how we look, what we say, and how we say it. NPs must enact the medical professional role if they are to be recognized as competent, in order to take on the clinical decisions traditionally held by physicians. This involves projecting the idea of control and objectivity that is inherent to the medical profession and is accomplished through a process of mystification, what Haas and Shaffir (1987, p. 2) termed a "special or transcendental authority." Mystification results from the use of certain symbols or rituals (such as abstruse language) that serve to reinforce the special and privileged status of those specially prepared to participate in their world. One such symbol of competence is speaking like a physician.

Learning to speak in telegraphic sentences and being able to look the physician in the eye while defending their treatment choices affirms the NP role and helps others recognize NPs' competence: "Without appropriate verbalization, how else would others know what you're thinking? Thinking can't be seen." Because the role is a moral one, it requires a drama in which players construct convincing performances of their special role, and in so doing both the audience and NPs are affected. Daily medical rounds are one of the main platforms on which the medical "script" is traditionally enacted and NP performance is legitimized by the audiences present. Being able to articulate and defend one's position when placed front and centre not only tests NP competence, but also allows for its recognition by the health care team. Recognition is subsequently validated and augmented when the physician publicly acknowledges the NPs' knowledge and skill. Affirmation helps to shape their emerging professional identity and their changing conception of a competent self:

It has been a huge bonus for us to be recognized and valued as collaborative members of the team. And when residents come into the unit or will be on rounds, the NP will often be valued and respected for their input as part of the team providing the care for the patient and family that day.

Patients and families also quickly recognize that NPs are deemed competent because they are placed at the fore in the time-honoured drama of being tested by the physician and on these occasions are heard to use the technical language of the medical profession. These practices elevate and separate them from the traditional nursing role and align them with medicine. Their ability to demonstrate their knowledge and skill to the satisfaction of the physician(s) during these times convinces not only the physicians but also the patients and their families that NPs are trustworthy enough to carry out the patients' clinical management at an advanced level: "And I guess it's because [the patient] would see me on rounds with the physician every day and I'd be there answering questions with the physician that she trusted me with that decision."

As one NP disclosed, NPs are perceived as competent when they speak strictly in problem-based terms; provide a running differential diagnosis; place the information into slots; identify the ways in which those problems can best be fixed; and then prioritize problems based on the whole picture. An outcome of developing competence is that NPs are better able to appreciate two key facts. The first is that in order to evaluate their progress in any particular case, physicians need NPs to present their clinical reasoning through their oral presentations. The second is that their oral presentations are effected by the contextual pressures of the acute-care setting; consequently, they need to edit information into bulleted lists.

Similarly, competence is revealed in the written language and form of medical progress notes and discharge summaries, two other privileged medical rituals. NPs' documentation, like their oral conversation, becomes disease-focused, targeted to the patients' chief complaints and related medical problems, and is concise and brief. Psychosocial information is integrated only when warranted, when it's related to the presenting illness or discharge plan. One NP said she had learned to condense case information to the point where she could do a history in half a page. NPs write what physicians want to know and, in so doing, communicate that they understand what is important to the physicians. Consequently, physicians interpret NPs' performance as being competent. Jimmy Santiago Baca's (1992) reflections offer insight into the power of coming into language:

> Until then, I had felt as if I had been born into a raging ocean where I swam relentlessly, flailing my arms in hope of rescue, of reaching a shoreline I never sighted. Never on solid ground beneath me, never a resting place. I have lived with only the desperate hope to stay afloat; that and nothing more.
>
> But when at last I wrote my first words on the page, I felt an island rising beneath my feet like the back of a whale. As more and more words emerged . . . I had a place to stand for the first time in my life. . . .
>
> Through language I was free. (pp. 6–7)

NPs recognize that they are the eyes and ears of physicians when they call to give them information; in this way, they help physicians visualize what they are confronted with. This situation is best facilitated when both parties speak a language that results in the same interpretation. Ironically, the expectation that NPs speak only in a manner that reflects competence as defined by the medical profession is gradually waived once their trustworthiness is established. In fact, when they are at a loss for the right words to describe what they are observing, they have only to acknowledge that "the patient doesn't look right" for their medical partners to respond to their requests for assistance. Actually, being unable to speak the language now becomes an indicator that an NP may be about to breach his or her scope of practice.

Regrettably, that recognition of competence, with its privileges of leniency, generally remains confined to the physician group and the health care professionals with whom NPs routinely work. It is not automatically conferred by others simply because competence is recognized and acknowledged in other publicly identified ways. Unlike those with an MD title, NPs must continuously prove their competence to each new member of the medical team:

> You look at the patient and since you know them you know the patient's sick . . . and the attending physicians just know if we say the patient's sick and we can't come up with the medical diagnosis that they need to come. . . . But we sometimes don't have the language that I think the residents need to hear, other than, "The patient's sick, he can't breathe. . . . I ordered this, this, and this. Is there anything I need to do?" And, then it'll be, "No. Call me when you get all those things back." Whereas the attending physician will come and see the patient, and say, "Yeah, you're right, the patient's sick. Yeah, we probably do need to admit him. Let's see what the X-ray shows."

Thinking like a physician refers not only to speaking like a physician, but also concerns bringing new knowledge to bear on practice situations where its application is problematic (Schön, 1987). Competence in clinical practice is demonstrated by the NPs' ability to independently initiate and make an individualized medical plan of care for a patient. In any given clinical situation (within the confines of their designated scope of practice) the NPs not only know that there is a health problem that needs to be addressed, but they also now accurately label the problems, understand their significance, identify possible solutions, articulate and defend the treatment plan, and take responsibility for implementing it, all with a diminishing sense of anxiety. Integrative system-thinking has become second nature when figuring out pathophysiological problems. They make multiple correlations in their minds in the form of running differentials and then narrow the range of choices based on the information at hand. They are able to do this on limited information, having learned to live with the risk of developing and initiating a treatment plan before having all the definitive information. Furthermore, many make their decisions under intense time pressures. NPs and members within their community of practice no longer doubt that their thinking process and skill performance can be repeated successfully under most circumstances. Perhaps being competent is most dramatically revealed when NPs replace the words *I don't know what to do* with *I know what needs to be done*, an outward reflection of an internal belief in their abilities to successfully perform independently.

> I mean, as you're training you're just learning and it's kind of like, I better call the physician on that because I'm not really sure what's going on or I'm not sure what to do. But now, for example, a child with hydrocephalus who's vomiting and very acutely ill with a bulging fontanel, I know what's going on and I know what treatment needs to be done. So I call down to CT and I say, "Can you squeeze in [patient] because he's having another episode." And I don't wait for the neurosurgeon to call back. I just know what's going on and then I just make the appropriate treatment plan.

Being competent means not only completing the newly acquired clinical tasks in an efficacious and timely manner, but also being able to anticipate future problems for both routine and dynamic non-routine events from a medical as well as a nursing clinical management perspective. Attempts are made to control problems by mapping out a plan of care, helping the team to prepare the environment, having the appropriate equipment and resources at hand, all the while fully realizing that the patient's actual presentation or responses to the interventions may very well alter these plans. The ability to do this, which Benner, Tanner, and Chesla (1996) illuminated as a major temporal shift in perspective in the novice-to-expert transition of staff nurses, is often the point at which an NP is able to say that she or he feels like a "real" NP.

Being competent is also characterized by NPs' ability to refocus quickly despite numerous interruptions; they discover that they are able to engage in multiple tasks simultaneously and can direct others without hesitation. They can hold in their minds information about multiple patients, with their complex issues and needs. They can delay some decisions without a pervasive sense of foreboding, knowing that the delay will not lead to negative consequences for the patient, family, or staff. This ability to prioritize demonstrates a shift that is integrally connected with conscious, calculated risk-taking. The number of patients that these NPs can care for efficiently and effectively has increased, so they are now left to manage patient care by themselves:

> I come in and check lab work on patients if I didn't have a chance to do it the day before. I'll look at what patients are being discharged that might need some follow up by me or make sure they've got prescriptions. Some patients might be going on Coumadin, so I need to look up what their INR was, call their GP, fax information to them, make sure the patient has a good understanding of what's going to happen for discharge. So that's done quickly. . . . Then I do rounds with the physicians and we determine who's being discharged, what tests or things need to be done. I try to get all those things cleared up before I go down to pre-admission clinic. . . . Down there, I do the medical or health history, do a physical examination, write the pre-operative orders. I tell them about what they're going

to expect when they come in for surgery. . . . Quite often the nurses are bringing me the lab results or chest X-ray results (from patients I've seen a couple of days before) and then I look at them to decide whether further things need to be done. Occasionally they need a CT scan to evaluate a nodule that might be on their chest X-ray or they might have a urinary tract infection. Some of them don't have family doctors so I follow up and come up with an antibiotic and fax or call that to a pharmacy to treat it before their surgery. . . . Occasionally there's an issue that comes up that I have to consult with the surgeon at some point, and I will jot those down and then deal with those at a later time. While I'm down there, I'm constantly being paged from the floor for issues that patients have, so whether they've got a low haemoglobin or maybe have some sort of a crisis that sometimes I have to come up to the floor and assess them and order ECGs, troponin levels, things like that too. . . . Occasionally, I might be assessing a patient for a knee replacement, but when I do my assessment I find that their hip is far worse than their knee, and so I change what orders are written. I talk to them that based on the X-rays that are done today we might be changing your surgery to a hip instead of a knee. So I'll do things like that too and then review it with the consultant at a later date.

When NPs demonstrate they can think like a physician, they are assigned call duties, another sign of affirmation of NP competence. Being on call means being the first notified by any health care professional to medically address patient-care issues throughout the weekday when the attending physician is present within the institution, or on nights and weekends, when he or she is not physically accessible. This act is, in effect, the physicians' public acknowledgment that they have placed their trust in the NP's level of knowledge, skills, and clinical judgments. It is what Turner (1969) calls a rite of reincorporation or reintegration (post-liminal) stage. At this point, NPs are brought back into the health care team and have an approved new status within it. NPs are permitted to belong, even if only marginally: "And if you've been here for a while the physicians trust you and so they don't necessarily come in and so I was responsible for these two small babies. There's nobody else there on nights, and so I got to do everything — put the lines in and make all the management decisions. It was the first time I felt like an NP."

NPs also receive affirmation of their competence through positive feedback, both subtle and explicit, from their physician colleagues. The words they hear not only lead to feelings of being valued but also validate their new way of thinking and acting. A more subtle, yet powerful, form of positive feedback occurs when nurses choose to seek answers to their clinical problems from the NP rather than calling the physician, physicians initiate a direct consult to the NP, and staff physicians inform new residents and their patients that they are to call upon the NP's knowledge and skills. Word of mouth within the medical colleague circle that an NP has the knowledge and skill necessary to care for a specialized group of patients is an equally powerful form of recognition of competence. For instance, an NP caring for a specific patient population with a relatively rare and complex disease process commented that general practitioners throughout the region recognized her capabilities by directly contacting her for advice on medical management issues for these patients. Similarly, an NP working in an infectious diseases subspecialty remarked that both physicians and nurses in the public health community across the province now directly referred patients to her and consulted her about their medical management.

Being competent arises from a certain degree of efficiency in the performance of skills, decision-making, charting, and communicating, and results in medical aspects of practice being gradually taken for granted. Now NPs begin to draw on their nursing background and actively integrate who they are as nurses into their clinical practice. They actively pursue the integration of thinking like a physician with thinking like a nurse. NPS incorporate nursing assessments into the medical history and physical exam, creating a more holistic health history. They not only decide what medication choices are available as part of the treatment plan, they free up time to explore these choices with the patient and family. After writing a prescription, they integrate patient teaching into their clinical practice. They have time to focus on the anticipation of future needs of the patient and family and can include long-term planning in their care management and integrate potential with actual patient-care needs, addressing multiple physical needs, including those associated with normal healthy living. For example, paediatric oncology NPS discuss potential sexuality and child-bearing issues with adolescent girls being treated for cancer, while cardiology NPS use the opportunity to explore lifestyle choices with patients and engage in health-promotion teaching about smoking, exercise, and nutrition once a myocardial infarction has been ruled out in the chest pain assessment clinic.

Being Confident

As NPS acquire more clinical knowledge and skill, they start to believe in themselves and believe that others trust them to do the right thing for their patients and families:

I've had to learn to say this is why I'm writing this and I know that this is right and move on. . . . I'm satisfied that I'm doing it right, it's correct, and nothing bad is going to happen. . . . The first time I felt like an NP was probably when I felt more confident and I felt I was doing a good job and was on the right track and things were coming together.

Little by little, feelings of self-doubt are replaced with self-assured-ness. NPs know and acknowledge that they are able to do what is required of them. They find themselves able to give timely responses to others' questions and concerns without the need to second-guess themselves. They do not constantly check their reference books or double- and triple-check their orders, nor do they need or want to verify every decision with a physician: "Three years later I would say that my confidence has definitely increased, so that for most diagnoses, I know what it is, I com-municate it with the parents and talk about the plan of care, and don't run back to the surgeon and double-check beforehand."

NPs' confidence is evident in their ability to discriminate between ordinary and unusual decision-making situations in their specific clinical practices without a pervasive sense of doubt or hesitation. In fact, they now describe parts of their practices in terms of the simple and mundane activities in which they are engaged: "By the time you've been doing it for four years, 90 percent of it is routine. So instead of it being 10 percent routine and 90 percent new, it's now 90 percent routine and 10 percent new. Even reasonably complex patients become routine because you're used to dealing with them." This sense of routine comes from an ability to recognize when one experience is similar to another. Such pattern recognition makes NPs feel more self-assured about their decision-making; a process that has been explored in great depth from clinical reasoning and clinical decision-making perspectives (Dowie and Elstein, 1988; Thompson and Dowd-ing, 2002). When NPs are confident, they say that with enough experience they are able to accurately pick out the common or normal sets of problems their patient population presents with. They differentiate between decisions that are easy because of their routine nature, despite complexity, and those that are dif-ficult because of complexity combined with newness or rarity.

Uremic syndrome is a biochemical entity and I can diagnose
hyperparathyroidism and I can diagnose hyperkalemia and I can
diagnose pulmonary edema and I can diagnose coronary artery
disease and myocardial infarction. . . . There's a lot of cardiovascular
problems, there's a lot of endocrine problems, and I'm comfortable
enough making those diagnoses and intervening, and beyond that,
I think they probably need a doctor.

This ability to discern what they know and not know helps NPs
to diminish their anxiety about the responsibility they bear and
their fear of causing harm. The times they feel disabled by their
responsibility becomes less frequent and intense over time:

Being scared is not as pervasive. . . . And I think I've developed
a certain level of confidence in what I know, what I can handle,
and also in what I can't handle, and knowing also, having worked
with the medical team for a while now, being able to say, 'Guys
I can't handle this. I'm going to take care of this patient but I need
back-up now.'

The pattern recognition associated with decision-making helps
NPs feel secure in their belief that they know, even in unfamiliar situations, the right thing to do. Although knowing what is
right is associated with being competent, it is also tightly woven
into their experience of being confident. This is evident in her
account of the first time "Jackie" felt like an NP. She described
numerous behaviours that were indicative of being competent,
such as quickly and accurately diagnosing the patient problem,
identifying how it needed to be solved, engaging in multiple
tasks simultaneously, and directing others without hesitation.
Her experience of knowing that she had taken the right actions
allowed her to feel confident and to finally identify with being
an NP. She accepted that it was permitted to not know everything

that had to be done or even whether the diagnosis was ultimately accurate. She no longer felt that she had failed the patient or that she was intellectually unable to make and act upon the appropriate clinical decisions. This was contrasted to a time in which her hesitancy, indecisiveness, and lack of confidence in the moment necessitated her calling the physician before she could act on her thoughts. Referring to herself as a novice in this situation, Jackie acknowledged that she had been unable to perceive herself as an NP despite titling, education, or others' perceptions of her competence. Being confident allowed her to experience being competent.

> And it was a woman who once again was having her first hemodialysis on an evening shift and I was working this shift. And she had just had a permacath put in . . . and we put her on dialysis, and she started going into acute pulmonary distress. And I listened to her lungs and I could hear nothing on the right side. And she had a diagnosis of Wegner's, which is an autoimmune disease that causes problems with both of the lungs and the upper respiratory tract, but I didn't think that was an adequate explanation. And so then I quickly thought about what are we doing to her on dialysis, and this is a new catheter, and I hear nothing here. And I wouldn't know very much about a shifting trachea but it looked like it [used her hands to demonstrate on her own neck]. So I wasn't able to intervene here, other than to stop the dialysis. . . . I asked the staff nurse to stop the dialysis — and I simultaneously ordered a stat portable chest X-ray and called the medical resident on call. And she had a hemothorax. . . . [A]nd it stands . . . in contrast to that poor unconscious lady my first evening shift in the unit where the very first thing I did was call the physician; whereas in this situation I had already made something of a diagnosis when I called the resident and I had stopped the dialysis. So I felt confident the right things had happened.

When they no longer feel disorganized, NPs do not automatically blame themselves for being unable to get everything done in a timely manner. Although time constraints continue to frustrate them regardless of their level of expertise, they are able to reflect on what is within versus outside their control to manage or influence. They identify when the workload is too heavy and will ask others to help them with their work. They admit to themselves and others what they have been unable to attend to without feeling shame or personal inadequacy.

> There are days where you may have seven kids to see in the morning before rounds; you might only see two, because when you got to number two, things were not good. And so then you've got to deal with the fact that you've got five more kids you haven't seen and you're going to be doing rounds and there's no way that you can get it done. I've learned now to say, like if the fellow is finished [with] his patients, I'll say, "Do you mind checking or mind going and seeing these?" I don't mind asking for help or just saying when we get in rounds, "I haven't had a chance to see this patient."

NPs discover that they know and trust their own instincts so they can dive into the fray easily and quickly; curve balls do not immobilize them in their thoughts or actions. They no longer need to mentally and psychologically prepare themselves for the problems they might encounter and have enough self-assurance to extemporize when problems present themselves unexpectedly, be they patient-related difficulties or those associated with working with an inexperienced team. "Betty" shared her story of one such curveball. She had been called to attend a routine delivery in which there were "a few fetal variable decelerations, nothing to really worry about." She expected that she might have to "just do a little drying and warming, maybe a little oxygen," but found herself in a full-blown resuscitation. She was partnered with a nurse who had never worked in this setting before and who questioned whether she should be replaced with someone more experienced. Instead, Betty offered praise and assigned specific tasks to specific team members. When the crisis was over, she publicly acknowledged that the situation went smoothly and, in response to the nurse's apology that she wasn't good enough, the NP gave her positive affirmations: "You were excellent," I said, "You did a really, really good job."

As their self-assurance increases, NPs take responsibility for patients with an even broader range of pathophysiological issues. Yet, because they now know what they know and don't know, and have more realistic understanding of the limits to their scope of practice and their responsibility within those limits, they also become confident negotiating the boundaries of their practice. Each NP articulates and defends his or her scope of practice for the specific clinical context and emphatically identifies for others what he or she needs to or should know. One NP laughingly said, "I don't do neuro" and "I've never put in a chest tube and I never will. I'm pretty clear about that." In other words, they confidently place boundaries around the knowledge and skills that they need in order to bring safe and timely care to the patients in their practices:

Some people think that they're responsible for the entire world and I don't ever try to assume that. I know there's one person doing that now and she'll always say, "But I don't know everything." I keep saying, "You don't have to know everything. I think you know what you need to know and now you have to be confident, be willing to admit when you don't [know] and seek help and guidance when you don't". . . . And so I know that I don't know everything and I know my limitations and then I'm willing to go out and do that.

NPS' confidence is influenced by others, particularly the physicians with whom they work and, when applicable, other NPS. For most, it is a continuous process of renegotiation in order to ensure that the boundaries created continue to be honoured. For example, "Nancy," who bore responsibility for performing tracheostomy changes, described this negotiation process. A staff physician new to their clinical team, having observed her practice, suggested that Nancy, not the ear, nose, and throat (ENT) medical resident, should be responsible for performing the patients' tracheostomy changes earlier than was Nancy's current practice. In this case, a change in the timing of the procedure amounted to a change in her scope of practice. She acknowledged her reticence about the request, recognizing that it was born out of knowledge of the deaths of two children during tracheostomy changes — despite having been performed by ENT specialists — before the stomas had been well established. Yet despite her reservations, Nancy was open to examining the various levels of evidence regarding patient outcomes, the additional training required to manage premature closure of the airway, and the system changes that would need to be instituted in order to safeguard the patients. As this example illustrates, NPS' confidence is demonstrated by their ability to recognize their strengths, link them to the salient issues in the situation and to ways of responding to the problems identified, and then bring them to the fore in the negotiation process.

There is, however, a paradox inherently associated with being confident: as NPS gain mastery of the clinical management component, they also enter new and uncharted waters as clinical experts. Tensions arise when they begin to surpass the expertise of their physician colleagues while at the same time they need their assistance when they find themselves outside their scope of practice. Struggling to do what is right for the patient and for one's self in the situation is clearly evident in the following account told by "Gordon," who encountered difficulties during the performance of a bone-marrow aspiration involving a very obese patient on whom he had performed a number of aspirations in the past.

> I did him with an eight-inch bone-marrow needle the first time. This time I couldn't reach him with an eight-inch bone-marrow needle. I was blind. And I called [the attending physician] and he was busy and he also said, "You're the most skilled of the group. You've done him all the way through." And as I was doing it, I thought, Yeah, I am. I agree with him. But I know the least about anatomy of them all. . . . I did it, but I thought, I am out of my league. . . . And I thought: What do you do? I mean, we're just not trained. And can we say, "No I will not do this procedure. I refuse?" Of course you can, but when someone says you're the most skilled of the lot, can I still say no? Of course I could have still said no but what I actually asked then was if they would mind me going to a different site, which they agreed that I could switch sites, just to do anterior, which they don't like me doing, but again they deferred to me as I was the most skilled, which is true. I've been doing the most in the last seven years. But it was an interesting position to be in. . . . And just as [the attending physician] was walking in the door, I got the specimen and it was good and everything was great. But the fact that he came down refreshed my faith in him.

As this example illustrates, being confident means that NPs acknowledge that they have a strong clinical grasp of the situation. They both recognize the familiar and individual patterns of responses and have a clear sense of when they are outside their scope of practice, based on the unfamiliarity of the clinical territory in which they find themselves. There is marked congruence between the confidence they express about themselves and others' expressions of confidence in their competence. In fact, both are even able to readily acknowledge when the expertise of the NP exceeds that of the physician in a particular clinical situation. Uncertainty arises when they know that they are outside familiar territory without the requisite knowledge required to legally engage in the activity. But the uncertainty experienced is different now than what they experienced in being adrift. Being confident results in an appreciation that they may have capabilities that others do not have, even when the demands of the patient situation may exceed their capabilities, and even when their capabilities may not be legitimately recognized in a court of law. Gordon acknowledged, "My insurance crossed my mind, and would they back me up?" NPs' recognition of the others' level of competence as compared to their own is then linked to the sense of timing required of the action for the sake of the patient and is quickly examined in light of other available options in the particular situation. All this information then culminates in a clinical judgment that is based clearly on a risk-benefit analysis.

While most nurses are able to turn to the cumulative and collective wisdom of their group for advice, the lack of a well-established homogeneous community of practice is strongly evident in Gordon's story. He described being so shaken that he approached a student in the NP program to talk about the event. However, the student herself was so overwhelmed with her own confusion that she actually asked Gordon not to discuss it with her. He contemplated discussing the experience with the nursing faculty where he had trained and with members of his professional association. Unfortunately, his previous experiences with these potential support systems had led him to believe that they were as much in the dark as he was when it came to NPs' scope of practice as it was actually lived in the practice setting. There were also no other NPs with his particular subspecialty in Canada whom he could contact at that time. "What do you do?" he said. "I didn't know who I was going to call." Two questions that are brought into consciousness by being confident and competent are held in the balance for pioneer NPs: Who bears the responsibility for the risk-taking associated with the decisions made at this level? Who is best to take the risk in each particular situation?

Confident NPs also begin to make the decision when not to act, that is, when not to over-treat. Being confident helps them "to do what is in the best interest of the patient, not what is safest for the nurse practitioner." They gradually find the fine line between being cautious and overly cautious, and see the patient that needs to be tended within a health care system. Confidence involves "not ordering fifteen tests when three would do because you have to consider the cost to health care." NPs recognize that they cannot always play it safe by doing everything all the time.

> And I don't think that people can take care of patients just by doing everything. And I tell people the hardest thing is not to do septic work on every baby. That's very easy. Every time they have a whimper or whatever I can send all the cultures off and start them on antibiotics. A much harder thing is to try and take all the information and say, "No, I don't really think it's an infection, this is something else." It's harder not to do everything. . . . There isn't a lot of good reason to do this except to make you feel good, or to think I'm doing something. . . . But if you stop feedings and start antibiotics all the time they just never make any progress. . . . You have to get to these points and you have to kind of make that jump: "No it isn't that and we're just going to progress and stay on with this course."

Being confident is also characterized by NPs intentionally holding off or delaying discussion of clinical management decisions with the staff physicians. Even when a clinical situation is outside their scope of practice, they believe that they can manage the event until the physician is able to assist them. In fact, they differentiate between keeping the attending physician informed (because the physician is ultimately responsible) and consulting a medical expert who can better deal with the issue or provide affirmation. "Donna," a neonatal NP, recalled how she had been summoned to the delivery room to assist the team with the resuscitation and stabilization of an apparently normal newborn after an elective Caesarean section. On arrival, she discovered that the baby's breathing was abnormal and the team was experiencing difficulty with intubation.

When I went to intubate him it just made it worse . . . [and] just all this stuff is going through your head — Well I know I'm going in the right spot, it's passed through his cords — but as soon as I do this it actually makes it worse, not better. I can give this baby CPAP and give him hand ventilation and it works much better than it does when I intubate him, so what is the problem? And so going through that and saying, "Okay, if this baby has a TE fistula then it can be that sometimes, once you pass the endotracheal tube, that you can go into the fistula and so that you have problems ventilating them or that you're hiding the fistula and all of your pressure actually goes to the stomach instead of where you want it to; it just depends on where it is". . . . So, I'll just continue with what is making him better, which is the positive pressure ventilation and maybe just the CPAP and let him do the work himself. He needs some help but I can't do it. So, I got the lines in quickly so we could monitor his blood gas and how he was doing, and I also phoned the neonatologist and said, "There's something really strange and you have to come in." And he wasn't really happy. He said, "Well, if you don't know, how am I supposed to know? Look, I'm not coming." I think I said, "You're probably right; we might need to call ENT for this; there's something wrong with this patient's airway; but I'm not sure that it's not just me."

Donna had a clear understanding of the normal patterns of response to an intervention and, as a result, readily acknowledged that she was no longer in familiar territory. Her confidence was demonstrated by her ability to use her knowledge and critical thinking skills in such a way that she calmly and quickly thought through potential diagnoses and possible actions. At the same time, she observed the infant's responses to the actions she employed in a trial-and-error format in this time-pressured situation. She continued to respond quickly and fluidly while managing multiple tasks. Even though she wanted to be able to do more for the patient and family, her skilled performance was linked with her ability to honestly assess her own capabilities. She called for assistance in a way that showed she now worked with the physician in a collaborative partnership rather than a hierarchal relationship. In this way, control of and responsibility for the clinical management of the patient was shared with the physician rather than relinquished. Even when she was unsure of one aspect of clinical management, she remained in the centre, directing what she could, complementing the work of others. Expressing a sense of failure was not about having failed as an NP because of ineptitude. Through the creation of a caring space for the distraught family, this information was even honestly shared with the parents:

> The family was up in the unit while we were trying to intubate and I described the procedure to them and then I had to admit failure and I said, "I've tried and it actually seems to make it worse, so, I'll just leave it as is, give him the help that he needs in another fashion, and I'm calling in these people. And what it says to me is that there's a very serious problem with the airway and your baby; we know that your baby's going to need surgery but I don't know what else to say beyond that."

Being confident also creates the possibility for advocacy and taking an ethical stance. If NPs are to be trusted to do the right thing, they need to perform in a way that is true to the intersubjective, social, cultural, and ethical concerns of the situation, rather than merely acting within a set of behavioural protocols or skills. It can be assumed, then, that the more thoughtful and reflective NPs are regarding a particular situation — calling upon all the ways of knowing that they have available to them — the more likely they will be able to act confidently in situations marked by contingency and uncertainty. Max van Manen (2002) regarded this as a quality of tact. For example, there is a moral imperative demonstrated in the act of acknowledging one's limitations in the situation and then insisting upon the involvement of medical colleagues, even when those colleagues argue against the need to be involved because of their trust in those very abilities.

NPs recognize the limitations of the abilities of medical partners in particular situations and take the risk to be independent thinkers despite the strong dependent relationship that exists. Donna described how, after she had verified her impressions of the case once the physician made his initial attempt at intubation, she was able to protect the baby from further ineffectual intervention and possible harm by physically intercepting and definitively stating the need for surgical intervention. She expressed a combination of anger and disbelief that he would not recognize or acknowledge his own limitations in the circumstance:

But unlike me he didn't stop. And I put my hand on his wrist and said, "He's actually better when you're not doing this. I think it's time to quit and then just make the referral. . . . We need to transfer him." So, he called the appropriate people and did whatever was necessary and it ended up the baby did have the most totally weird airway in the world; it was really non-operable. . . .
So, the challenge was the decision-making for the neonatologist:

"You've got to quit now because you're just making him worse. This is exactly what I have done; I'm satisfied it wasn't just me, but now we have to call in somebody else."

In due course, NPs learn to create a façade of knowing so that even when they do not have a full understanding of the intricacies of the situation — the anatomy, physiology, or pathophysiological process — they are still able to exude a sense of confidence in their ability to safely handle it. They thus embody the medical aura, a phenomenon described in the medical literature as "a cloak of competence" (Haas and Shaffir, 1987; Merton, Reader, and Kendall, 1957). Ironically, this cloak is not developed or used by NPs until they have confidence. When confronted with uncertainty, they don the cloak in order to communicate the impression of competence and confidence, of being in control of the situation: "People tell me I know everything. I know I don't know everything, but I must present this aura of confidence. I just don't tell everybody I don't know everything. I need to have some confidence so that people can trust what I'm going to do and they'll listen to what I have to say."

NPs accept that members of the team expect decisiveness and action, action that is taken in a calm and inclusive manner: "The nurses want you to be able to make a decision. In a crisis, they want somebody who knows what they're doing and doesn't fly apart. . . . They do say that some people just kind of fall apart in a crisis and that's not very useful or that they just boss them around and they don't really want that either." The consequence of controlling and manipulating others' impressions is that NPs increasingly identify with their role and become even more confident. It would seem that there is a quality of self-fulfilling prophecy in these authoritative performances that contributes to a changing self-perception. Dr. Glenn Colquhoun's (2002) poem When I Am in Doubt expresses the power of this façade:

When I am in doubt
I talk to surgeons.
I know they will know what to do.

They seem so sure.

Once I talked to a surgeon.
He said that when he is in doubt
He talks to priests.
Priests will know what to do.

Priests seem so sure.

Once I talked to a priest.
He said that when he is in doubt
He talks to God.
God will know what to do.

God seems so sure.

Once I talked to God.
He said that when he is in doubt
He thinks of me.
He says I will know what to do.

I seem so sure. (p. 89)

Learning to project confidence is part of the medical mystique. How NPs present themselves to nurses, physicians, patients, and families is as important as the content of that presentation. In an occupation that demands such a great measure of trust from the health care team and their clients, NPs must convince audiences of their credibility. They quickly realize that the audience looks for cues and indications of personal confidence. In response, they orchestrate a carefully managed presentation of self intended to create an aura of self-confidence so they can affect the patient's medical plan of care in a positive way:

> You've got to have confidence. If you present your plan of care as,
> [slowly, softly, hesitantly] "I think and maybe perhaps", then the
> person listening to you is not going to or might not trust you as
> much as, [boldly, loudly, and quickly] "Well, I think this and so
> my plan is to do this." Take out all the perhapses and state your case
> and be prepared to defend it. Don't defend it unnecessarily because
> then they'll think — well, you're not really sure. So, it's a whole
> way that you present yourself to the world.

An aura of confidence is facilitated when NPs learn the routine ways of treating a particular problem or the acceptable patterns of therapeutic interventions, along with the likes and dislikes of the various physicians with whom they work. Nevertheless, even after years of experience, they still sometimes experience uncertainty about how a particular physician will think in a given situation. Yet, they are able to retain the illusion of confidence by speaking definitively about parts of the plan of care while being vague about others. They open up discussion in a way that allows them to discover the physician's thinking during the debate, so they can maintain their input into and control over the final decision. As one NP shared, "Even though you make your plan out and you order the things that you're sure of, the things you aren't sure about you learn to keep your decisions nebulous and to keep those things for the general discussion on rounds and then you say yes or no to them."

Accepting that they can never be completely right all the time, while realizing that they can always learn from each experience to make a better decision in future, is part of being confident. NPs accept that they live in a grey area in which they "could do this or that," and have learned to make a choice without waffling while being confident that neither decision will cause harm to the patient. Making a decision is almost as important as being able to make the best decision each time, the latter gradually appreciated to be an impossible task in many situations.

NPs nonetheless experience times in which their confidence eludes them. For example, others may still intimidate them, particularly some physicians. Specific clinical situations may cause them to doubt their ability to perform. "Alex," with more than a decade of experience as a neonatal NP, described how attending deliveries for newborns with meconium aspiration still fills her with self-doubt, making her uncomfortable and apprehensive:

> It's in situations where you think that's a weakness of yourself perhaps, or somebody that can intimidate you. I never like going to resuscitations where there's meconium because then you have to intubate their trachea in the case room. They're all slimy; it's [a] completely uncontrolled [situation]. And so I was called in the middle of the night to this delivery for this baby and everything that could go wrong went wrong. And I'm kind of that little — you know, if I had to evaluate myself I would think I was not so sure of my skills in that area — so when everything went wrong and the physician who was there said, "What's your name?" And you're there thinking, "Oh, you're not happy with my performance! [aggressive tone] How long have you been doing this job?" [laughs] So yeah, I wasn't very confident there. . . . It's easier to feel non-confident.

Although these situations may not cause the same intensity or duration of doubt and apprehension as they did at first, NPs continue to work hard to reduce the gaps in their clinical knowledge and skills. Feelings of insecurity serve as the compass for more knowledge, which leads to continuous learning and growth:

> I'm kind of that knowledge person and I try to erase the deficiencies so that I do know what I'm talking about and that I'm sure of it, so that I can be confident. It's when I'm not exactly sure. But I think as you do the role more and more, then . . . if it's something

that doesn't require immediate decision-making, I'll say, "Well, I'll just read this because I can't recall the exact details but I'm going to go look it up and then I'll get back to you."

To summarize, in feeling competent, NPs believe they know how to do something, have the power to make things happen, and that their efforts will be successful. They exhibit confidence when they complete the task at hand and "just know" that they have done well. They have little doubt about the outcome of their perform-ance and need no external feedback. Ironically, being confident increases the likelihood of a task being performed well because it enables people to make the most of their abilities (Davidhizar, 1991, p. 105). The union of confidence and competence in the NP role now makes being comfortable possible.

Being Comfortable

[He] learned what it meant to leap into the void . . . [Plot-ting a meticulous route on the nautical chart] had been a source of satisfaction in a profession where accomplishing safe passage between two points situated at far-spread geo-graphical latitudes and longitudes was essential. There were few pleasures comparable to deliberating over calculations of course, drift, and speed, or predicting that such and such a cape, or this or that lighthouse, would come into view two days later at six in the morning and at approximately thirty degrees off the port bow, then waiting at that hour by a gunnel slick with early-morning dew, binoculars to your eyes, until you see, at exactly the predicted place, the gray silhouette or the intermittent light that — once the frequency of flashes or occultations is measured by chron-ometer — confirms the precision of those assessments.

When that moment came, [he] always allowed himself an internal smile, serene and satisfied. Taking pleasure in the confirmation of the certainty achieved through mathematics, the on-board instruments, and his professional competence, he would prop himself in one corner of the bridge, near the mute shadow of the helmsman . . . content that he was on a good ship, rather than in that other, uncomfortable world, now reduced by good fortune to a faint radiance beyond the horizon. (Pérez-Reverte, 2001, pp. 33–34)

So for most things, I'm comfortable that I can make the right decision. And if I'm unsure, there's always someone to call, always. You're never a boat alone in the ocean. It's somewhat like sailing around in a marina.

During this period of being comfortable, NPs feel like they have finally come home. The word *comfortable* means to be in a state of mental and physical ease, to be free from hardship, pain, and trouble (Barnhart, 1988). When "at home," NPs are at ease, comfortable with themselves; they are able to be who they truly are. They experience feelings of relief, pleasure, enjoyment, gladness, and even transcendence in their work. Although a sense of awe, wonder, or incredulity with discovering what they are capable of is now rarely experienced in their clinical practice, smooth sailing in the harbour is a preferred place to be at this point in their journey. In the novel *The Unbearable Lightness of Being*, Milan Kundera (1984) examines the question — "Which shall we choose? Weight or lightness?" (p.5). While Kundera acknowledges that, although "the heaviest of burdens crushes us, we sink beneath it, it pins us to the ground" (p. 5); he suggests that "the heaviest of burdens is simultaneously an image of life's most intense fulfillment. The heavier the burden, the closer our lives come to the earth, the more real and truthful they become" (p. 5). Perhaps then, being comfortable is revealed as a weightiness of being that occurs when NPs believe their practices have meaningful substance despite the heavy burden of responsibility. Their clinical practice is no longer experienced as burdensome but rather as a source of deep satisfaction.

Initially, being comfortable is experienced as a bodily perception, indicating that NP's practice is becoming easier. The mental fatigue previously caused by moment-to-moment decision-making is no longer evident, and in its place there is a taken-for-granted feeling that their clinical work is second nature: "I can remember being just so mentally tired from making these decisions and then I can remember not being tired. I can remember a call shift and I wasn't tired and it was just so easy to make decisions. . . . It was just a couple that were difficult, that you had to really think about. At that point I was [thinking], 'I can do this.'"

As a result of renewed energy, the opportunity to enjoy learning resurfaces, and clinical problems are perceived as a series of opportunities for being stretched and challenges to be faced with a sense of excitement:

> I think every day is [a good day because I actually learn something new] when I'm working in the unit . . . I don't get bored with my job because there's always something new . . . it's always changing. . . . Even in the field of cardiac surgery in this new era of stenting and [performing] multiple procedures in the cath lab, it's changing the environment of surgery, because now . . . we're only getting the ones that they've tried everything else on for the last ten years. . . . It's exciting now; it was scary then.

In fact, once knowledge and skills have been honed, some NPs hanker after more challenging clinical situations, wanting to continue to push the boundaries of their abilities. This sense of wanting to be stretched re-emerges as an aspect of being comfortable. Feeling scared is no longer a state of being but rather is accepted as an integral part of the excitement of risk-taking. One NP, for instance, felt comfortable enough to recommend to her medical colleagues that she establish and manage an independent clinic of a particular subspecialty patient population within their larger practice. She derived great pleasure bearing that responsibility.

Because NPs have become more efficient and effective as individual practitioners, their teams become more efficient and effective too, and NPs and team members no longer think about the momentum of the day. This sense that a service or program runs itself implies that the team trusts each member to know how to do what is required of them, at the performance level expected, and they respond to each other in a synergistic manner; team members come together in the enactment of their practice only to be strengthened. Thus, team comfort serves to enhance NPs' feelings of comfort:

> I think we've settled into a lull . . . settled into a good system. . . . It's nice now; it's just comfortable, to the point where, if I'm out of town, [the physician] will say people don't know why he's come to do the procedure instead of me, because they expect me to be there. . . . It's now more taken for granted. . . . Now it feels like our team runs like a well-oiled machine and . . . nursing is very much a part of that running of the well-oiled machine, to the point where we don't wonder why things run so well anymore, because they just do.

Settling into a routine helps NPs create boundaries or a comfort zone, an internal safety line, within their scope of practice. The comfort zone is the internal place where feeling at ease is experienced and results from engaging in work in a way that requires less effort and distress. In this zone, the earlier pervading feelings of uncertainty fade from the NP's everyday awareness. Little by little, uncertainty (and dealing with it) becomes integrated into NPs' lives such that it no longer requires active management, nor is it experienced as solely distressing. Uncertainty has gradually evolved into a certainty in their strength and resilience. Kolcaba (2003) spoke to the ability to rise above the discomfort of uncertainty when it cannot be avoided or eradicated as *transcendence*, a type of comfort that speaks to comfort's strengthening property. In fact the word *comfort* also means to strengthen: the words roots are *cum* which means "together," and *fortis* means "to be strong" (Barnhart, 1988).

Certainty is encouraged by physicians; they are quick to admonish when uncertainty is displayed, indicating that doubt will impair their effectiveness with patients. In fact, Katz (1984, pp. 184–206) has suggested that medical socialization involves *training for certainty*, not uncertainty. In this state of being comfortable, even uncertainty takes on new meaning. NPs realize that many of the decisions they make are not white or black; there is a wide grey area, an area of differences of opinion and a variety of choices that may lead to similar outcomes. Some choices may be better than others, but not all choices are necessarily wrong or bad. Although this helps to diminish the fear associated with the responsibility of clinical decision-making, it creates a taken-for-granted tension between certainty and uncertainty: "I know the more I learn about making those decisions, I realize that there's no right or wrong either. . . . It's not as exact a science as you think it is." The reality of needing to initiate a plan of care before all the definitive information is available contributes to this understanding that choices made may be less than perfect or even wrong.

So much of what you do initially is based on scanty information. . . . [E]ven in the end, you may not have enough information to say for certain . . . but you have to just take this limited amount of information and say, "I think it's this, this, or this, and then this *is how we are going to manage each one." Maybe there's conflicting ways to treat them so you're going to have to make a decision — "Well, I really think it's this." And I mean you're going to be wrong sometimes but other times it's kind of where the clinical and the laboratory and diagnostic information leads you and the patient, and it kind of changes, and I'm comfortable with that now.*

Being comfortable means that NPs also accept the certainty of their own imperfections, yet they accept the responsibility of caring for fragile and vulnerable patients, knowing that the choices they make can cause harm and even death. They have learned to live with the internal struggle to be perfect in the direct clinical-practice component of their role: "I guess I recognize that you can't be perfect. This job makes you realize that. You have to be humble because if you think that you know everything and that you are always right, you won't survive, because we all make errors; we all may make not exactly the best decision at the time, and you have to deal with that." NPs are the first to acknowledge that they do not have the same breadth and depth of knowledge as physicians; yet they are also quick to acknowledge that medical knowledge itself falls short — a lesson first learned as a bedside nurse and then reinforced as an NP. Being comfortable means that a balance is found between being sufficiently decisive, certain, and in control, and recognizing the uncertainty that abounds in what they do. It does not mean that they wear what Katz (1984, p. 198) has referred to as the medical "mask of infallibility" so often worn by physicians.

The tension between uncertainty and certainty leads NPs to continuously strive to provide the best possible quality of care by reflecting on their mistakes, never taking for granted the decisions they make, asking for help when necessary, knowing when they are outside their scope of practice, and reducing knowledge and skill gaps through constant learning. In spite of this tension, they come to terms with their need to be perfect, for without doing so, they either stifle their own practice opportunities, preventing timely responses to patient care, or they live with a constant anxiety that not being perfect brings to bear.

And some of us deal with it very well; others of us get way too uptight about it, and it doesn't benefit our families for us to be so constricted that really we're not working at the NP level but we're still at the bedside level. Or the other issue is to become so blasé about it that you just think, Oh well, it'll all work out in the wash, and then something happens and it doesn't.

Even the need to create an aura of effortless perfection, the mystique that is often associated with the medical profession, finally gives way. Obviously effortless perfection is an oxymoron; the illusion of perfection requires an enormous amount of work. This is one reason for the sense of exhaustion that new NPs feel when they are trying to prove to others and themselves that they can do this job. They are elevating medical perfection to a high art, but perfection, as Quindlen (2005) wrote, eventually becomes "like carrying a backpack filled with bricks every single day. . . . What is really hard, and really amazing, is giving up on being perfect and beginning the work of becoming yourself" (p. 11).

The NPs' ability to do just this while performing in their new roles is truly difficult and amazing. It is difficult because it means others may see that NPs do not always know what to do in the clinical management of the patient and so may reject or replace them, both as individuals and as a practising group. But this ability is also amazing because letting go frees a person from having to work so hard, all the time, to pretend they can know everything concerning their clinical practice. Ironically, letting go of trying to be perfect frees NPs to accept more responsibility and undertake more risks. The tension NPs have learned to live with is accentuated for two more reasons. First, there is no NP zeitgeist to guide them. Second, their previous grounding in a nursing moral imperative necessitates that they reject the mask of medical infallibility that they were compelled to put on as part of proving they were clinically competent:

[Responsibility] can be exhilarating at times and it can be almost disabling at times, because all it takes is one instance for you to second-guess yourself, to say, "Should I have done something different, would I have done something different if I had known this or that or the next thing?" Or [for] a physician to say to you, "Well, did you think about such and such?" and to think, Well, yeah, I did but I discounted it; but should I have thought about it more? To think, This is too much; I'm not a physician, I shouldn't be doing this; this is way outside the scope of practice, when in actual fact it's your own sense of well-being and perfection that's getting in the way. And then to be able to say, "No, I did the best for this child and this is how it worked out and maybe it's not what anybody else wanted but this is how it worked out." And those moments make you think, Okay, I just want another job; I just want to be doing something else, I don't want to be doing this. But then, all it takes is one of those families to turn around and say, "I'm so glad that you're on the other end of the phone and that you could answer my question". . . . And you learn from those areas where you had some doubt and where you think, Okay now I'm going to do such and such. . . . And then other times you just have to say, "Bad things happen" . . . and you didn't, in all of your ego, have as big an impact upon the outcome as you thought you did.

Although being comfortable means that uncertainty is generally a taken-for-granted experience on a daily basis, various circumstances, such as managing a new clinical event or a change in the medical team — especially if it involves the loss of a trusted physician or the addition of a new member — brings uncertainty into full awareness, with the full range of emotions that this evokes. One NP described the surfacing sense of unease that came with a change in medical directors in her service. She was once again faced with the awareness of uncertainty as to how she would acquire her patients, the population to whom she would be assigned, and the expectations regarding her role under the new medical management. However, she discovered that this sense of unease, resulting from uncertainty, was also embedded in being comfortable with her own clinical competence and confidence. She felt a sense of certainty that she would eventually be able to negotiate her way through this situation to the satisfaction of the patients and families, the physician, and herself. One can observe her sense of relaxation with the negotiation process and the timing it requires, as well her patience and adaptability to the clinical situation, in the following quote:

> With our previous medical director, I was very comfortable with how I acquired my patients and whether I kept them or not. This current cardiologist is brand new to the system; he's brand new to practice, and so he and I have a few bugs to work out. . . . With the previous medical director, if I said to him, "This family has these issues," he would say, "Do you want to take them on and I'll see them in your clinic time?" Whereas this particular cardiologist doesn't necessarily like to be there during my clinic time, which is a bit difficult because then he would have been more comfortable with me keeping more of what he classifies as the complex patients. . . . And so he says, "Well, those patients need to get seen but I want your surgical patients and you take those routine non-surgical cases." So, I think we'll do a bit of negotiation over the next couple of months in order to get that worked out, because my background is surgery, that's how I started as an NP was to do cardiovascular surgery. I don't want the families to lose my expertise for them,

because they need the time and they need the expertise of somebody who's been in the operating room, who knows what the repair looks like, who can tell them what the post-operative period is going to look like. They need those questions answered. They're not going to get that from the cardiologist.

Uncertainty also arises when NPs are forced to acknowledge the tenuous nature of the medical safety line. As explored in chapter 2, "Being Adrift," the presence of a safety line is integral to NPs' clinical practice in an acute-care environment. A lack of confidence in this line brings about an awareness of uncertainty so powerful that it brings into question the entire foundation of NPs' clinical practice. If they cannot trust their physician colleagues, they are unable to trust the decisions that they themselves make, and consequently they question the ethical nature of their practice. At one level, this crisis is not dissimilar to that described by Benner, Tanner, and Chesla (1996) at the stage when competent nurses learn experientially that seasoned health care providers make faulty assessments or treatment orders, which undermine their confidence about the authority of these colleagues: "In reality, these nurses are confronting both incompetence in some co-workers and a necessary correction of their inflated expectations of experienced staff" (Benner, Tanner, and Chesla, 1996, p. 101). But at another level, there is a significant difference relating to the degree of responsibility that NPs bear. They often do not make the initial primary admitting medical diagnosis in the acute-care setting, yet they are responsible for ordering the treatments associated with it. Their role in the patient's outcome is therefore both more attributable and visible as they set into motion a set of prescribed activities that will either help or harm the patient. There is a sense not only of guilt by association but, even worse, a feeling of being an accessory to their medical colleagues' poor performance. In other words, they are reliant on the competence of their medical partners and the physician's will-ingness to engage in self-reflective practice and make personal or systemic changes to decrease patient risk and promote safe prac-tice. Physicians have repeatedly expressed their concerns about potentially being held liable for NP errors in practice. The ques-tion arises, *Should this not be a reciprocal concern for NPs?*

"Sheila" shared her experience of having discovered first-hand the fragile and illusory nature of her safety line. She was once again living daily with the dis-ease of uncertainty despite having developed a strong sense of confidence and competence in her clinical abilities. Because of her profound discomfort, the meanings that constituted and sustained her practice as an NP were crum-bling. Sheila no longer experienced being clinically comfortable:

I verified with the doctor that day that this was in fact the right protocol that this [patient] should be on and reviewed the orders. . . . Well, lo and behold, the next day the [physician] who had picked that protocol realized that it was the wrong one, and in fact [this patient] could die if we continued to give him this treatment. . . . And you know, I almost died as well, because I had seen [the patient] that day and regardless of whether or not I had signed those orders — I hadn't been the individual to sign the orders, although that was definitely a factor — I had a feeling like, What's going on here? Can I not trust my physician colleagues to pick a proper protocol? I almost signed those orders. If that [patient] had died from this protocol, my name is on those orders. I don't want to lose my nursing licence over a situation like this, and probably more importantly I feel that you have to be able to look a patient in the eye and have them feel that they can trust you. And that was starting to waver for me. I wasn't sure of myself anymore, or my colleagues . . . and it just came to a crisis for me . . . in terms of the NP role and thinking that I'm not sure that I like this role anymore, and what I'm doing in it. . . . What do I need to do

*to feel comfortable going to work every day? What is my role in
relation to all those protocols? . . . If I'm going to be signing orders
and admitting [patients] under protocols, I have a responsibility
to know those protocols, right? But I don't pick the protocol either;
that's the physician's point. And I'm just trying to sort through all
of that in my own head right now. What I do in the NP role, I'm
not sure about anymore . . . and right now I'm feeling overwhelmed
with . . . the weight of that responsibility and feeling like, What if
I can't trust everybody on this team? What if there is one individual
who I'm having some concerns about in terms of their practice
and . . . the thoroughness of their work?*

Sheila's story demonstrates the profound tension felt when NPs
are again confronted with the stark realities of their own vulnerability within their practice. It serves as a persistent awareness of
existential uncertainty and the tenuousness of the NP role. It had
taken her nearly five years to reach the point where she could
say, "This is a bit routine; I am feeling comfortable with this
aspect," but only a split second to lose it. This supports Cohen's
(1995) theory that particular triggers can heighten the awareness
of uncertainty, which in the case of NPs causes them to question whether the work demands are worth the personal cost. It
also demonstrates how one's identity is closely linked with a loss
of being comfortable due to the resurfacing of the awareness of
uncertainty, as experienced through engaging in action with one's
community of practice. Sheila explained her need to take a break
from the clinical component of her role because the physicians
had chosen to ignore this and other patient safety concerns. She
acknowledged that there are no guarantees that mistakes will not
happen, but she expected everyone to think about the issues and
try to put into place the changes needed to diminish the risks.
An internal battle involving the social and ethical nature of her
work is revealed. At this point in her journey, she is experiencing

difficulty in reconciling the form of membership she has with her medical colleagues and struggling with who she is in this role.

In understanding what it means for NPs to lose their safety line, consider Pi Patel's experience of surviving a storm at sea only to come face to face with the loss of his life raft in Martel's (2002) Life of Pi:

> I noticed the loss of the raft at dawn. All that was left of it were two tied oars and the life jacket between them. They had the same effect on me as the last standing beam of a burnt-down house would have on a householder. I turned and scrutinized every quarter of the horizon. Nothing. My little marine town had vanished. That the sea anchors, miraculously, were not lost — they continued to tug at the lifeboat faithfully — was a consolation that had no effect. The loss of the raft was perhaps not fatal to my body, but it felt fatal to my spirits. (p. 253)

Recall Gordon, who found himself in new and uncharted territories as an expert in the performance of bone marrow aspirates. He experienced a crisis related to the uncertainty he felt when he realized that his skills had surpassed those of his medical colleague, while at the same time he still needed this colleague's support. Gordon felt greatly relieved when he saw the physician's face and realized that he was going to back him up. This relief reveals the uncertainty that he must have experienced, even if only momentarily, and illuminates the faith or confidence that NPs have in the presence of the safety line. Physicians' presence helps NPs to overcome their dis-ease by providing a sense of being heard, a moment of being together, of not being alone in difficult situations. As a result, they re-experience a sense of well-being, or, as Buytendijk (1961, p. 21) eloquently wrote, "The stream of life within us seems renewed or strengthened." In contrast, Sheila is experiencing a crisis of faith in the foundations of the safety line; her uncertainty arises from the limits of the collegial relationship on which she is dependent.

The loss of being comfortable, experienced as a state of dis-ease, is the awareness of uncertainty that is attributable to outside forces, that is, to those who potentially or actually impact negatively on NPs' work. This awareness results in a sense of responsibility for having caused actual or potential harm to patients, what Cassell (1992) has called "paranoia" in her study of surgeons. Is it possible that the more dis-ease some NPs feel as a result of a sudden awareness of uncertainty, the more likely they are to publicly project these feelings onto others in a disparaging way, not unlike surgeons? Is it possible that this is one outcome of becoming visible? Now, the outcome of a clinical event, whether positive or negative, occurs before an audience and is attributable to the NP; both the NP and patient know who is responsible. Certainly, Cassell attributed these two factors to why surgeons are so aggressive not only in what they do but also in how they interact with others, particularly when it involves actual or potential errors.

In the following passage, an NP describes her reaction to a near-miss encounter that occurred during an operative procedure she was performing. Although she recognized that her reaction to the nurse's error may have been excessive and hurtful, she also revealed the fear and doubt she experienced when she was suddenly faced with the depth and magnitude of the responsibility she carries. She was made aware, in a particularly public venue, that she could possibly have perpetuated the mistake of another, which would have resulted in the patient's death. Not negating the influence of individual temperaments, perhaps the need to make the incompetence of the nurse visible was also in part due to the performative aspects of NPs' work. Now that the outcomes of their actions are both more attributable and visible, perhaps some feel a need to critically judge others publicly, or as Cassell

(1992, p. 181) suggests, "The public glory of victory is balanced by the fear — and shame — of public defeat."

We had a new nurse who thought she was being helpful and delivered the drug that's being given to the [procedure] room to me; and I was just about to start the procedure and she came running in the room and said, "You forgot the medication upstairs," handed it to me, and I just glared at her. And I don't think I'm really a mean person, but she just started to cry and cry, that's how I looked at her, because that's the drug that's killed some patients, and she brought it down. I had one of the nurses in the room call upstairs to warn everybody that she was on her way back upstairs, because I didn't even say anything. But however I looked at her was enough for her to just melt into tears and start crying because she was handing me a drug that I could have given that would have killed the patient. I mean hopefully I would have checked it and I would never have given it but just that, like that tells you how the fear and . . . [long pause]

In summary, NPs experience being comfortable when they are strengthened through ably doing, acting in association with a trustworthy safety line, and being recognized by others for their abilities. But NPs must also perceive a fit between their expectations for clinical practice and those of others, not just in terms of clinical competence, but also in terms of the type of practice in which they wish to engage. They convey being comfortable through such terms as *being excited, having fun, being satisfied, feeling safe, being happy,* and *having found the perfect fit.* How they embody their practice is as important as what they do in their practice. At home in their practice, feeling most like themselves, they are able to relate to others in the way that is most meaningful to them and that they experience as making a difference. What differences do NPs make in their clinical practice? This is revealed in being committed and being connected.

Being Committed

Acting skilfully, being present in the moment, listening, providing information, reassuring, explaining, and exploring the meaning of the illness event with the patient and family are integral to NPs' practice and to their sense of identity in their role. They are committed to the personalized care of the patient and their families, which is enhanced by being competent, confident, and comfortable.

The word *commit* is derived from the Latin word *committere*, formed from the roots *com*, meaning "to join with," and *mittere*, meaning "to send," as on a mission, in the form of a function or service to humankind (Barnhart, 1988). In this light, being committed means NPs are entrusted or charged with the safekeeping of those they care for. They must connect themselves to Others and, by implication, dedicate themselves morally to their cause. Being committed and being connected become interrelated in their practice.

Being committed speaks to the NP's desire to provide ethical care by being with others in the moment, in a context of doing for others within their clinical practice, and is an expression of their caring as nurses. It is strongly demonstrated in the intentionality of their actions, in the meaningful and purposeful personalized care of patients and their families from moment to moment. Indeed, throughout NPs' narratives there is a strong sense of commitment, of responsibility and accountability to the Other. Commitment is an act of will, a desire to do what is believed to be right and good in each moment, in every situation, despite the risks or burdens. This is well expressed by the poet Rainer Maria Rilke (1975): "And if only we arrange our life according to that principle which counsels us that we must always hold to the difficult, then that which now still seems to us the most alien will become what we most trust and find most faithful" (p. 99).

Integral to being committed is being technologically competent. Nightingale wrote in 1899: "The artful nurse knows more
than what is to be done; she knows 'how to do it'" (quoted in
Johnson, 1994, p. 7). Being technically skilful is a matter of pride
for many NPs, as well as an expectation of the role in acute-care
institutions. "Well, I do like doing procedures. It sounds like I'm
bragging but I'm extremely skilled," said one NP. The ability to
perform skilfully is primarily judged by self and others in terms
of such criteria as proficiency, efficiency, and fluidity (Johnson,
1994). Yet many NPs respond in each situation with an intention
to treat the patients holistically. Why has there been little or no
appreciation in the discourse for this? Do we fail to see or reveal
it because technology as care is not valued?

At one level, being skilful is about technical mastery and
receiving immediate gratification for a job well done. Having
achieved the desired outcome while making everything look
easy and with a natural rhythm, speed, and flow is a source of
great satisfaction. Positive feedback comes in a variety of forms,
from being recognized by one's colleagues as an expert to being
sought after by patients and families to perform a procedure.
For some, being technically proficient is about being in control,
being able to take action (however risky) rather than standing
by and waiting for others to act. For a few, there is also a "love
for doing skills." The thrill that comes from having successfully
engaged in high-intensity technical procedures in which the
high risks associated with failure are great is at once terrifying
and addicting: "I love to do the initial resuscitation. Some people
say it's the adrenaline rush. . . . Yeah, you're terrified a lot of the
time. But when you get it, it's like, 'Oh, I did it, I accomplished
it. This is such a great day.'"

In a profession in which external rewards are few and value for
what nurses do is generally unacknowledged (or sometimes cred-
ited to the broader medical profession), the success of undertaking

technical aspects of the role is so satisfying because the rewards are immediate and the victory is rapid, definitive, and ascribable. One NP stated that the hope of using technical, advanced techniques was one factor that initially drew her to critical-care nursing and then to the NP role. When asked to talk more about this desire to perform procedures, she responded, "I think it's a very concrete thing in nursing. . . . With technique, you go to put in an IV, you take that catheter, you put it in, it's in; that's the immediate reward. And I think in nursing we don't have that many immediate rewards. . . . It's challenging, it's sometimes difficult, but yet it's very rewarding."

The significance of the instrumental nature of the role as a means to visibility is also revealed in the following NP's thoughts. She described how satisfying it was for her to be able to perform percutaneous intravenous central catheter (PICC) insertions throughout the hospital. However, she felt equally frustrated at being blocked by physicians in performing other procedures in her practice — procedures she knew NPs did as well as or better than physicians, based on documented evidence.

Whenever there is a patient that needs a PICC line in the ICU, we will be involved in inserting it, plus anywhere else in the hospital, which is quite new here. And so it is nice developing some clinical skills that, in the NP role here, we've not been allowed to do, you know, inserting art-lines, inserting chest tubes; it's really not part of our practice at all. In the unit, the docs are not open to that yet. . . . They say, because we're in a teaching hospital, every resident and fellow that comes in wants to do technical stuff. So we're never involved in any intubations. Never. It's not even discussed.

Being able to engage in highly skilled functions is a gateway to professional advancement and autonomy, and to cultural authority and visibility. When NPs are obstructed from engaging in the instrumental functions traditionally aligned with the medical realm and highly valued by society, the credibility of the NP role as one of independence and authority is undermined. This creates doubt and confusion in the public's mind about the very nature of the role. Patients and their families have difficulty accepting the role or the person in it as valid or trustworthy.

> Well, you meet with the family, you explain to them that you're doing an important job, that yes, you're a nurse but in an expanded role. And you're with them and you develop a relationship and then whenever something happens, you've been pushed aside because somebody else is going to take over, so your credibility may be challenged in the face of the family. . . . Whenever something happens you're not skilled enough to do it, so maybe what you expressed before wasn't right, right? So we claim we're doing continuity of care, and we make a claim in face of the family that we're as knowledgeable as anybody else on the medical team, and then whenever something happens, you're suddenly not skilled anymore. So we're put in a difficult situation.

Since the emergence of NPs in the United States in the 1960s, the discourse has asserted that NPs are differentiated from other nurses, in large part, by having expanded "their use of medical instruments and the use of instruments in ways previously denied nurses" (Office of Technology Assessment, 1986). The personal autonomy, authority, and visibility this has afforded have been contentious and viewed unfavourably by many in the nursing profession (Harding, 1980; Purnell, 1998; Sandelowski, 1997, 2000). However, this discourse and the stagnant view of NPs as junior doctors who relieve physicians of medical procedures that they find boring has devalued the possibilities for caring to emerge in each patient encounter. As Locsin (1995, 1998) contended, when procedures are viewed merely as technique there is a degeneration of what it means to practice. Rather, an encounter between the NP and patient holds the possibility for discovering new ways of caring as a result of NPs' being in control of the performance of the medical procedure itself. NPs in this study did not deny that they often feel frustrated that a large part of their practice is spent performing medical procedures, under time constraints that limit their opportunities to engage in a patient or family encounter, which would allow them to get to know them on an individual basis in the way espoused by the philosophical tenets of nursing. Yet despite the challenges they face in this regard, they integrate a caring intentionality into their performance that improves the overall well-being of their patients and their families. Indeed, NPs' stories challenge the assertion that they nurse the technique rather than the patient, as implied by Sandelowski's statement (2000, p. 189) that the NP role "has reprised the one-nurse-to-one-technique, as opposed to one-nurse-to-one-patient, model of nursing care."

Recall Donna's story about the difficult intubation, presented in the section *Being Confident*; this NP's narrative revealed the possibility for advocacy and taking an ethical stance different from that of medicine. Donna intervened when the physician was unable to admit that he could not successfully intubate the infant with the TE fistula. She protected the baby from further ineffectual intervention and possible harm by physically intercepting and definitively stating the need for surgical intervention. Thus, when the NPs' instrumental function is viewed in a deeper way and within the full context of their practice, it is possible to elucidate their nursing identity and the moral imperative that they bring to bear on the procedural event itself. Indeed, the ultimate goal of their performing clinical procedures is a desire to improve practice for the good of the patients and their families. NPs recognize and accept that the use of technology is a reality of acute-care nursing in Western society. There is an undeniable tension created among the NP, technology, and patient. Nor is it denied that some NPs may act simply as technicians, proficient but not authentically present with their patients. Because of its frequent association with providing cures, technological competence does not have to be polarized against competence in providing care. In responding to the patient's call, NPs are in fact ethically required to be technologically proficient, while accepting the patient fully as a human being, not as an object (Locsin, 2001).

For many NPs, advocacy, as it relates to the instrumental nature of their practice, arises from a fundamental difference in the training of nurses and physicians. In nursing, one NP said, learning a procedure is all about the patient, while in medicine it is all about the skill. This is demonstrated in medicine's philosophy of "see one, do one, teach one" (Merton, Reader, and Kendall, 1957), a mantra that causes many NPs a great deal of unease. However, this has less to do with being afraid of performing the technical aspects of the procedure and more to do with wanting to prevent negative outcomes that result from ineptness, and to appropriately manage any adverse events should they occur. It concerns doing what is both right and good for the patient while performing the skill. Hence NPs ensure that their medical colleagues are present or near at hand until they feel ready to accept the responsibility of performing the procedures on their own, even at the expense of being perceived as overly cautious. "Grace," for example, shared her experience of learning to remove an arterial-venous sheath, a skill that she felt was not mechanically difficult but carried the potential for significantly adverse cardiovascular events in about 15 to 20 percent of people who have a sheath removal:

I think [physicians] were in the mindset of the medical student — see one, do one, and teach one — which is not my way of doing it. I wanted to be sure that I was doing these things really to the best that I could do. . . . The harder piece is the assessment of the patient to be sure that they're ready to have the sheaths out . . . and then managing . . . the cardiovascular complications. . . . Because of where the femoral nerve runs, when you're compressing it, a lot of patients will have profound vasopressor syncope. Their pressures will fall to nothing; they'll lose consciousness. Some of them will seize . . . which isn't great when you're holding an artery and this person's seizing. . . . So you can get somebody with a heart rate of 70 or 80 go to a heart rate around 30 and their blood pressure will go from a 120 to 60 by palpation and they're losing consciousness, and you've got one hand on their groin . . . I mean that sounds bad enough, but it's even worse if they've had an interventional procedure because the perfusion pressure through the artery, if that drops, then the artery will collapse and then they'll infarct because it's a raw area. So it's critical that that perfusion pressure doesn't drop. So learning to manage that, being able to detect it quickly, being able to give the IV atropine, often multiple doses of pressors, tons of fluid, as well as monitoring them for vascular complications in the leg. . . . And each patient is different. . . . So when I was learning the procedure I did the usual — watched a few and did quite a few under supervision . . . and after a while they said, "Okay, we'll just go and wait at the nursing station and if you need us we're here." So there was a gradual weaning and I was probably ready to do it long before I let them go. But it was just more my feeling that I wanted to be comfortable because when I was doing it on my own, they were scrubbed in the lab, so if there was a problem they weren't able to come and help me. So I had to be able to manage anything that happened myself.

For NPs, technological competence as caring is not just about mastery of the skill; it concerns being constantly attentive, vigilant, and prepared to respond appropriately, swiftly, and deftly in the event of danger, distress, or deterioration in the physiological functioning of the patient during the procedure. This means that they need to know what to look for. But as Hawley (2005) recognized, knowing what to look for is not as simple as it seems:

> Vigilance requires a sound and integrated knowledge base composed of theoretical (scientific) knowledge learned through study (e.g., pathophysiology, clinical manifestations, diagnosis, treatment, and potential complications), practical knowledge gained from experience (e.g., typical clinical trajectories or "the normal course of events" and known risks or complications in specific patient populations and subpopulations), and particular knowledge of the patient, including the clinical facts (e.g., co-morbidity or co-existing disease and injuries) and knowledge of the patient as person. (p. 181)

The NP's intention is to do good (Algase and Whall, 1993) and be fully present for the patient. It may be argued that technology can be rendered safe in the NPs' hands only when they are adequately prepared. Entering the world of the Other is coming to know the Other as a person more fully through the competent use of technology (Locsin, 1998), which most likely does not result from the educational philosophy of "see one, do one, teach one."

Being committed, as embedded in technological competence as caring, is also reflected in the NPs' need to know the intimate details of the technical apparatus and to know the patient in relation to technology. More specifically, the patient can be considered safe only if NPs acknowledge the impact technology can have on the patients' care, both positive and negative. This happens in the context of knowing a particular patient and family in the moment.

The other day, there was a bedside nurse who was busy with something else and she asked, "Can you take over?" and I said, "Yeah, I'm sitting here anyway so no problem." So a few minutes after, [the physician] came and said we need to give this and this. . . . Now, where should I give it? No idea. I didn't know the lines; this is really technical but I didn't know where I should give that without taking any risk. So I said I wouldn't do that. I didn't know that patient; I also didn't know why we needed to give that medication, because I was just coming in and I didn't have the time to know the patient, and I didn't know what was the family's understanding of the situation. Is there anything else that I should know on this particular patient? And I felt really pushed because I didn't get the background that justified that medication. I thought I was able to take over but I was missing information.

Knowing who the patient is in relation to what is required in the way of technical care is an essential element of NPs' commitment. Knowing the patient's and family's wishes emerges within the NP–patient relationship, during which the Other's world opens up to the NP (Boykin and Schoenhofer, 2001). In this view, the skill is not considered mechanistic but is revealed as humanistic and interconnected; care being provided by NPs is not based upon the evidence-and-cure process, in which their functions are narrowly described as the diagnosis and treatment of disease and the ordering and implementation of instrumental interventions. Rather, their use of technologies becomes an expression of caring and commitment. NPs have in fact, brought the Other into the right relation with technology.

The NPs' capacity to make a humanizing difference in their patients' experiences of technological events is what Hawley (2005, p. 130) has termed "combating the technological imperative." NPs express moral discomfort in situations in which physicians get "swept away" (Tisdale, 1986, p. 429) by the use of technology in the fight to cure at all costs. At the same time, they also experience discomfort when technology is withdrawn or withheld if little regard has been given to the patient's voice. Either situation represents a "lapse of humanity" (Frank, 1991, p. 27) in the face of technology. But NPS view their role as an opportunity to better influence decision-making within the health care team by illuminating the human values that are embedded in each situation.

We have one patient right now who is terminally ill with multiple myeloma, and who has had quite a bit of pain, and whose family and just about everybody thinks he should stop dialysis. But I was pretty sure that the patient didn't think he should stop dialysis then because I asked him about it on more than one occasion. He has a 90-year-old mother and he doesn't want to die before his mother; he thinks that's too hard. He's a quiet man and you have to sort of pull it out of him, never married and has siblings who love him and are very good to him. But the family was really struggling with this, so we decided to have a family conference. . . . I think they saw this meeting as a chance to develop a plan to bring him home for palliative care to a little town outside of here. And I said, "Okay, but we have to have the patient here because I'm not certain what he wants." So I started the meeting and I asked the patient what he wanted. And he didn't say anything really because he's this quiet 70-year-old bachelor. So, I said, "I'm going to push here because everybody's here because they want to know whether or not you want to continue dialysis, and if you don't, we want to begin to plan to get you home so that you can enjoy some time with your family in your old home." And he was ambivalent; I know he was. . . . And he finally said, "Well, I guess maybe we should plan." So we planned, but it was a Friday and we knew we weren't actually going to be able to get the plan implemented and talk to [community services] until Monday. And by Monday he had changed his mind. And I actually feel badly about that. I hope we didn't coerce him, but the important thing was that everybody then realized that [he] didn't want to come off dialysis.

By establishing a relationship of intersubjectivity, NPs are in a key position to speak out on behalf of the patients. Because of their involvement over time, they come to know the meaning of the health care event in the context of the person's experience as whole. As a result, they develop an ability to sense from the patient's perspective where the boundary between harm and benefit lies (Gadow, 1989). This engaged knowing enables NPs "to speak, not with their own voices, but rather, to the extent possible, with the voice of the patient and in so doing truly fulfill their moral responsibility to foster patient autonomy" (Hawley, 2005, p. 133), what Gadow (1989) has argued is the hallmark of true advocacy. Similarly, NPs reveal their capacity to make a humanizing difference in the experiences of their colleagues caring for people who are suffering and dying. In taking the time to help others reflect on patient choices, to respond in a manner that reflects attunement to and genuine concern for the predicament of others who are sharing the patient's life as lived with the choices made (e.g., nurses), NPs further demonstrate their commitment to Others.

Because he looked so awful, and because it's such a big unit, even if it's in the chart, you have to retell the story over and over and over again, and you have to help the family who are still struggling with the same issue, which is he's literally got skin over bones and the pain has continued to be an issue that we've struggled with. So, just helping everybody be clearer . . . that it's time to stop asking this man whether he wants to continue and just get on with his goal, which is to continue dialysis and to have pain relief. So I'm often sharing that, particularly with the staff nurses, because I mean they struggle. You know, they're spending four hours with him and I'm spending fifteen minutes with him twice a week. But I talk with his family about twice a week and I've talked with the social worker and I've talked with the community support people who were continuing to come back and check . . . so, just making certain the plan of care is clear and everyone is supported in supporting him.

For many NPs, the desire for more control over the instrumental aspects of practice is not driven by a personal need for external validation as an NP. Rather, it concerns the acquisition of control of the procedure to better enable nursing both to meet an individual patient need and to more positively impact the broader care delivery system. Being committed is demonstrated in seeking opportunities to provide holistic care in a more timely and effective manner. Much of patients' and nurses' time is spent waiting for physicians' availability to perform a procedure, resulting in unnecessary discomfort, increased anxiety levels, and discharge delays. Frequently, patients wait all day until physicians are finished their surgical cases or clinic appointments to interpret an X-ray, insert or remove a chest tube, or administer an intrathecal medication.

"Grace," the NP who undertook the removal of arterial-venous sheaths after angioplasty, emphatically expressed that an NP's approach to practice should not be about what the physicians or nurses need; rather, the question driving NP practice should be *What are the needs of the patient that are not being met that the NP can assist with?* As Grace noted, timely removal of the sheath brings greater patient comfort and autonomy and reallocates nursing care to others: "It's how you can best meet the needs of the patient, and if it means you take knowledge and skills from traditional medical functions, that's okay."

[Patients] can't get out of bed with these sheaths in; so, they'd be ready in the morning to have the sheath pulled but the physicians didn't pull them until four or five o'clock in the afternoon. Patients

were on bed rest all day when they could have been up walking around and be using the bathroom by themselves rather than the bedpan. . . . The work load for the nursing staff was huge because these patients are on bed rest and have to be monitored with these arterial sheaths. . . . So that was the first thing I said: "Okay, this is the need; that's the first thing in terms of skilled focus that I'm going to work on."

Commitment to patients and their families is also revealed in the tensions that some NPs experience when they assume some of the technical aspects of practice that have traditionally been held by physicians. The burden of the instrumental nature of their practice, in terms of either the responsibility carried or the belief that the goals and ideals of nursing are at odds with the increasing demands directly associated with technology (Locsin, 1998) is negatively experienced. However, their commitment to the provision of holistic, continuous care intercedes. This commitment grows stronger when they are in relationships that feel powerfully connected or when they are acknowledged and appreciated by the patient and family to be a trusted care provider.

I don't really mind doing the procedures when I look at it from the perspective that the families really appreciate me doing them. Yeah, it's a medical technical skill, but I mean everybody has that in terms of their job. Nurses have got to put in catheters and do all kinds of stuff. I mean, there's that piece of our work, right, and that's basically how I view the LPs, because it gives comfort to the families actually to know that I have an expertise in that area, I can do it quite well, and they know me very well and they trust me with their loved one and this particular painful procedure. So I don't really have a major problem doing that. At first, I wondered: How will this go? I'm not sure I want to do this, that kind of thing. But when I looked at it from continuity of care, the families do really appreciate me doing it.

Being committed to technological competence as caring is an ethical dimension that NPs embrace; they are committed to use themselves in relation to instrumentation in such a way that they can physically or emotionally strengthen their patients and diminish patients' and families' anxieties or concerns.

> I like kids not to hurt. . . . It's been three years of hard work to get to the point where I am; that we're not scrounging up screaming kids and hurting them. So that's part of the joy is just that now we do them . . . with no pain. . . . We have a treat box and give them all sorts of things and a [child-life worker] works with me to get them into the room, and a team of anaesthesiologists that help me sedate them, and then the technicians who take the specimens. I love to get good specimens and get good slides. . . . I like the guys in the lab to report "excellent specimen" because then I feel like I've done the best possible job that I could and that the child doesn't have to go back to sleep again for another one. And . . . doing the best possible needles to the least headaches that you could ever have. . . . So, just to be able to do it once, in just one shot, and no band-aids, just shoot it in. And I'm arrogant as all get out. I like to aim it in and never miss and to get clear fluid with no blood. Yeah, it's pure joy to do a perfect procedure.

At first blush, the proud and audacious nature of this description is striking — the NP's ability to identify her own strengths, the confidence she has in her own skill. It is reminiscent of surgeons' arrogance and certitude and their surgical motto, "Sometimes in error, never in doubt" (Cassell, 1992, p. 175). There is also a sense of competitiveness vis-à-vis her performance, a striving to be perfect. But, on closer examination, there are other layers associated with being committed to a technological competence of caring. First, performing the diagnostic procedure well makes a repeat procedure unnecessary and the findings more reliable.

Second, being able to do the procedure perfectly also means that patients will experience less discomfort afterwards, and adverse effects will be minimized. But this NP has also embraced the performance of the skill from a holistic viewpoint. By embracing the procedure, she embraced the opportunity to change the philosophical approach to how patients were cared for, thus revealing the moral agency of her NP practice. Seeing an opportunity to change the way in which the children were sedated for the procedure, the NP seized the opportunity to work with a large interdisciplinary team to initiate a procedural program that took the developmental needs of the children into consideration along with the pain and sedation management issues. A choice of pharmacological approaches, enhanced with hypnosis and play therapy, was part of the program. Connecting with the children through demonstrations of tenderness and caring during the performance of the skill were also evident in unique ways: "I put nail polish on them when they're asleep. . . . I learned how the boys appreciated it because they were bright silver and [one boy] even went out to [a] party with them silver." As embodied in technological competence in the form of caring, being committed is revealed when NPs demonstrate compassion, conscience, competence, confidence, and comportment. The stories shared by NPs reflect their capacity to give beyond the practical significance of the act. A generosity is demonstrated in "the skilled touch, a seeking contact with the person as much as it seeks to effect the task" (Frank, 2004, p. 6).

Being committed, particularly as it relates to NPs' involvement in the instrumental nature of their practice, is also revealed in their willingness to accept and reflect upon their failures and mistakes. The intent of their reflection is to modify their approach, in order to provide the best care they can to their patients during the procedures. Although being comfortable and confident means being at ease and experiencing a sense of routineness in their work, NPs do not become unconcerned or blasé about the responsibility they bear. The mere fact that they have stories associated with past mistakes and then choose to recount and reflect upon them during the interviews demonstrates their need to express their concerns and anxieties. The retelling is a means of reaffirming that they continue to be caring persons in highly technical environments. These stories are ethical ones, and they are another means of revealing the commitment and existential caring embedded in NPs' clinical practice. "Joseph" shared a story about an event involving a technical procedure in which he attempted to cannulate an umbilical artery even after several attempts by another colleague. This experience shaped who he was as an NP. It was a difficult story in the telling, even years later:

> And so I should not have tried that one more time. Did that make the difference? Did I cause the complication because of my obsession to get this intervention done? So living with the consequences of that was tough. I mean the child did fine but . . . you know, I was the last person to have tried the line and I probably should have just respected my colleague's call on it and let it go at that. . . .
> It's tough to know when to stop, when to recognize your limitations, and then living with a decision that you made that had consequences. And it's more than just personal self-reflection. What have I done with it? It's made me a better nurse in terms of respecting when my colleagues say that . . . they've given it their best shot and, unless I'm invited to have a try at it, be respectful of their decisions. Knowing when enough is enough and not being afraid to say, "We can't do this anymore to this child." And then . . . going to the mom and saying that this was a side effect of an intervention that we were trying to do to your son was a humbling experience in itself. . . . So that affects how you give information to parents later on down the road too. So in many, many different venues it influenced my practice.

Joseph dwells on his story even many years later. This is in Heidegger's (1971, p. 147) sense, "to cherish and protect, to preserve and care for." This story implies value (Frank, 1995), and in sharing a story about a mistake he made, Joseph calls us back to what is ethically significant: it was not enough only to reflect upon the reasons for his failure to do no harm, he also had to take the lessons learned and enact them so as to protect and care for others in the best way possible in the future. His story reveals the vulnerability of patients and their families and the NPs' responsibility toward patients during the performance of a procedure, the need to do things for the right reason, and the need to respect and extend the strengths of colleagues on behalf of their patients.

NPs respond to the call of the vulnerable who need them to act "responsively and responsibly" (van Manen, 1991, p. 97). Nightingale (1992, p. 11) wrote, "A careful nurse will keep a constant watch over her sick." But to watch over, or be vigilant, requires that the caregiver demonstrate a commitment to knowing the Other. In an attempt to know the patient better, NPs intentionally acquire a greater depth and breadth of knowledge and skills, to have these at their command in the actions of caring not as a substitute for caring, but as an enhancement of caring. Activities such as interpreting data from laboratory and diagnostic tests, observing patient's responses to the manipulation of various therapies, and then engaging in an ongoing interpretive quest (Leder, 1990) at an advanced level are legitimate ways to know the patient whose needs have intentionally called the NP to action.

Attentiveness to details (via knowing and sharing them), being familiar with routines, and continually scrutinising the broad spectrum of technology for pieces of information that helps them know the patients better are all ways by which NPs demonstrate their commitment to being vigilant:

> One day a resident commented to me, "Oh that's funny." And I said, "What do you mean, that's funny?" And I was doing fluid orders, so I went to the patient, looked at the pumps, looked at the different IV accesses. And he said "That's funny" because the resident would sit at the desk and would .try to do his best but without ever looking at the patient. I said, "Come on, it's IVs, medications are going to the patient, I need to look at them." And he said, "Yeah, yeah, yeah," but he would look at the chart, and maybe ask the nurse, but he wouldn't look at the patient. And I thought, Yeah, but maybe that's a good difference [between being an NP and doctor]. We'll look at the patient, we deal with families, and we sit with them, we spend time, which may be different than what the doctor will do. Yeah, that was funny. Just fluid orders, it's nothing, but you know the patient is getting the fluids.

There has been an assumption that by knowing the patient biologically in a deeper and broader way, the NPs' focus of care will be reductive and objectified, resulting in the traditional series of problem-solving actions that are embedded in a medical model of care. Yet NPs demonstrate that to know the patient's physiological status in the moment, or which life-saving or life-enhancing treatment options to offer, based in a focus on commitment, is to be connected with the patient. They are then challenged to respond authentically and compassionately as an advocate for the patient in the moment and in the particular. This requires that they know each patient fully as a person.

"Mrs. Jones" was a woman living with an inoperable neuroendocrine tumour. Her husband had brought her to the oncology clinic because he had found her generally unwell, with intermittent fever and confusion. With the concern that her cancer had metastasized to the brain, she was admitted to the hospital for follow-up tests under the care of "Helen," the NP.

The very afternoon she came in, I reviewed the orders they had
written in the clinic, and they forgot about half of her meds, so
I had to do that. Then I went to see her, and the nurse came to me
and said, "By the way, her temp's 39.4." And this lady is usually
very talkative, very vivacious. She's 73; you'd never know it. She's
involved in all kinds of women's things, the women's institute, and
she's hardly ever home when you call her. But she was not well.
She was curled up in the bed, very withdrawn and didn't want to
talk, and you could tell she just didn't feel well. Anyway, I said,
"Well, they're saying that a lot of what you're experiencing could
be drug related" — she's in a clinical study because her cancer's
progressed on every other therapy they've given her, so she's in this
trial and some of this could be related to the study drug itself —
"however, let's do blood cultures."

Although the last thing anyone had expected was that Mrs. Jones
would have an infection, because her white count was normal,
Helen was able to call on all of what she knew personally about
Mrs. Jones to make the decision to test for other possible reasons
for her behaviour. In so doing, she avoided closure. She did not
abandon the search for the cause of Mrs. Jones's symptoms in
favour of the logical and predetermined rationale. Being attentive
to all details of the situation, including scientific, instrumental
knowledge, Helen was able to discover that Mrs. Jones was sep-
tic. Knowing this particular patient in a qualitatively distinct way,
combined with what she knew to be the normal presentation of
patients with sepsis, Helen was able to intuit a problem that was
incongruent with what one might typically expect in the situation. She immediately initiated the appropriate life-saving medical
treatment of intravenous antibiotics. Within several days, Mrs.
Jones was feeling better, and Helen began to initiate discharge
planning. Her vigilance helped to keep Mrs. Jones safe from harm.

In addition, Helen observed during this admission that Mrs.

Jones's husband was quite nervous about taking her home. He was concerned that no one was paying attention or doing the right things for his wife prior to her hospitalization. Acknowledging that much of what she did as an NP was to help her patients and their family members feel safe to return home, Helen felt charged with a duty to reduce Mr. Jones's feelings of anxiety. First, she ensured that home visits for physiotherapy, occupational therapy, and nursing care were organized upon discharge. Then she worked with both husband and wife in such a way that she could assist them to cope with the emotional crisis they were experiencing:

> What we were prepared to do was to LOA to discharge, which we don't do very often. . . . I said, "What we can do is we can give you a leave of absence tonight, and you just call in tomorrow, and if the night goes well and there are no problems, then you just call the nurse's desk and say I'm staying home and then you'll be officially discharged." . . . But in fact the husband wanted to leave it until Saturday. I said, "Well, let's see how it is tomorrow morning" and the wife said the same thing. . . . So I went in the morning prepared to say, "Okay, we can be flexible. It'll be either today with discharge tomorrow, or Saturday to Sunday," and he said, "No, I think it's fine. I can see that she's a lot better and she's getting better by the day, and why take up a bed when I'm sure you have other people who need this bed and with health care dollars being what they are."

NPs embody being committed by being present for their patients and families, by hearing their concerns and responding to them in a way that is inclusive and egalitarian. They know and use the system in a way that offers patients creative options that help reduce the chaos they may experience during the illness event. They do not seek closure to the relationship simply because the physical problem has been solved, but take responsibility for all the issues to ensure that patients do not fall through the cracks.

Being Connected

Because of the nature of acute care in today's health care system, many relationships with patients are intense and of short duration, yet NPs are committed to development of a relationship with patients and their families; it is about *being connected*.

The best part of my day is actually sitting down with the mom or dad and just hearing their stories and trying to understand this crisis that they're in from their perspective. . . . For many of our families, it's the first time that they've ever had to deal with a crisis of this magnitude, so, outside of all the other resources — the social worker and our CNS — as a nurse practitioner, what else can I do for this family to try and put all the pieces together and keep it together and identify what their needs are? That's the best part of the day.

NPs often struggle to find the time to make connected relationships that they find satisfying and sustaining on a daily basis. The rapid turnover of patients, their responsibilities for providing clinical management for all of the patients, and the families' preference to seek information directly from the physician may interfere with their ability to get to know the patients and their families such that they feel connected in deep and meaningful ways.

As an NP, when you talk to the families, it's more an information-giving session, a question-answering session; it's not as much of a one-on-one, get-to-know you kind of thing, unless the patient's there for a significantly long time and then you get to develop that relationship over time. It's just because you don't have enough time at each patient's bedside. Sometimes I struggle with that whole thing because if the patient's family wants information, they often want it from the doctor. . . . And a lot of families don't even know what an NP is, for starters. So you have to try to develop that relationship

*and say, This is who I am, and This is what I do, and I'm
always around, and If you have any questions or you
want to talk about what's going on with your family
member, I'm here for you. And I like to get to know them
on a one-on-one basis, but it's not always possible, and that part
I really, really still feel a significant need to try to improve.*

Yet despite their struggles, NPs experience profound moments of
connectedness that occur through showing respect and sensitivity
to the patients' and families' needs; talking to, listening to, and
being honest with them; being available by encouraging them to
call if problems arise; and appreciating them as human beings.
"And I always give them my business card and I say, 'If anything
happens, if you have any questions, or you start feeling unwell
again, I'm on my pager. You just call me.'" One NP used spare
moments in her week to contact four or five of her patients just
to say, "Hey, how are you doing?" simply because they appreciated it. Another said that the most personally satisfying time in
the day was when she was able to create even a few moments
with a patient to "just sit there and chat about their garden." Even
such simple but respectful and generous acts as personalizing
care by referring to the patient by name rather than by diagnosis and bed number, and the use of spatial arrangements, opens
the opportunity to connect.

*The cardiologist stands, the NP sits down. I say, "Well, come into
the quiet room . . . come sit here and we'll talk about this," and
that's very different than what they're used to. They're used to a
cardiologist coming in and standing over top of the echo bed and
standing there while they're sitting. They get to ask a few questions,
he answers and then he says, "I need to see you in such and such a
time," and then he goes away.*

Simply put, NPs believe that patients and families want to be heard and attended to. They embody the belief that "an important component of healing, apart from the effect of any technology applied, derives from the relationship between the healer and the patient" (Matthews, Suchman, and Branch, 1993, p. 973). Being connected with the Other begins in the welcome and the opening of self to the Other and is a form of generosity. As Frank (2004, p. 2) has noted, "Generosity begins in *welcome*: a hospitality that offers whatever the host has that would meet the need of the guest."

NPs have a profound respect for the value of connectedness and the comfort that it provides. Being connected is their promise not to abandon the Other. It is a struggle for them to sustain their moral commitment to the patients and their families when they are continuously challenged to battle the physicians' commitment to medical education, fraternity, and an orientation of disease. One NP spoke about the time that she arrived for medical rounds only to be informed by the attending physician that she would not be needed in the clinical area because of a surplus of residents scheduled for the month. Although her initial reaction was one of shock and disbelief, she immediately connected with the patients and families for whom she had been caring to explain the situation. She was concerned that they would feel abandoned by her and believe that she had not valued their relationship. But in attempting to smooth the transfer of the patient's care from herself to a new medical care provider, she recognized that the change was going to cause unnecessary suffering:

And I went to the family and said, "As a team we're . . . giving your care to a good resident who will be really good with your son, really good with you, and . . . who will continue what we've been doing with you." And it might have been my mistake to accept the staff physician's decision, but she started to cry and said, "No, you cannot leave that way and leave me alone with all my problems, and it's not going well, and at least one thing is that we've got continuity and we've been really happy to see you on a daily basis. No, you cannot leave that like that."

In response to the this implicit question *What am I to do?* — what Frank (2004) described as a microethical moment — the N P subsequently chose to follow through with her commitment to the patient and family by successfully defending her need and right to remain a part of the clinical management of the patients and families with whom she had been previously involved. This story is not about the N P arguing that she provides better care than the physicians or her fight for a de-marginalized position in clinical management because she had been blatantly declared superfluous; rather, the mother's reaction to being "handed over" crystallized for the N P the essential moral commitment that she carries in that role. "Holding to the difficult" (Frank, 2004) in the interpersonal, locally contextualized, moment-to-moment, she chose to fight for the right to remain connected because she understood its therapeutic value.

N P s' effectiveness is based on relationship-centred caring with the patient, their families, and sometimes even the community (Watson, 2008). For many N P s, their patient and family relationships involve much more than treatment of disease. They attempt to establish relationships that respect patients' and families' values, knowledge, and skills, and give their voices as much authority as their own. Being connected in this way is the difference between speaking *about* and speaking *with*; it invites patients to be open and honest about their health concerns and struggles. This in turn provides a fuller picture of the patients' situations and allows N P s to make accurate diagnoses and fashion individualized management plans. By collecting data about various aspects of the patients' lives, N P s are able to understand health and illness concerns from a wider perspective than that of a list of medical diagnoses. This understanding allows them to be more effective in meeting the patients' true concerns.

A few physicians have said to me, "Oh you're thinking like a nurse again," as if it's a bad thing. And I don't take it as a bad thing. They're thinking more — what's this person's immediate health problem? Let's solve it, and then off you go on your way. And they don't really take into account the rest of the patients' lives and what's going on with them. . . . Whereas now I like to know more about the people and more of the social aspects than just the actual medical base . . . because I think it all plays in. I mean oftentimes when we have patients — the very sickest ones that have to have a continuous intravenous infusion of Flolan, which is a pulmonary vasodilator — all they can do is walk around with this little cassette with this infusing constantly. And quite often a couple of them will come in with headaches and say, "Something's wrong with my Flolan." Well no, they've had a fight with their son. So it's the other things in their lives that are going on that [you learn] if you just sit there and talk to them. And I don't need to change anything medically because there's really nothing medically wrong. So I think it's just as valid as dealing with their medical condition.

By encouraging patients and families to discuss the biographical and social contexts of their lives, NPs empower them by maximizing their voices. As an outcome, the asymmetry so common in the medical relationship is minimized. According to Fisher (1995), "It is this combination of medical and psychosocial skills that differentiates nursing from medical practice and that grounds nurse practitioners' claim for professional autonomy" (p. 9). Many NPs understand that patients balance a unique set of commitments and obligations, such as work and child care, which determine the amount of energy they can bring to caring for themselves or their loved ones. Each individual has a personal history of successes, failures, hopes, dreams, and fears that shape how he or she responds to the illness event. Each patient presents with varying cognitive and reasoning skills he or she uses in self-management of his or her condition. Each patient has unique values, beliefs, and goals regarding how he or she chooses to live. NPs know how important it is to understand each patient's strengths and weaknesses, values and beliefs, fears and goals, when negotiating a treatment plan that will optimize his or her health.

There's one individual who's had HIV for quite a number of years and he's Muslim. . . . He used to come in and we would figure out from the lab tests that he hasn't been taking his meds even though he says he was. . . . And for some reason we developed a bond. I spent about two hours with him one day and we talked a lot about religion and spirituality. . . . He was interested in kind of where I was coming from and I was interested about where he was coming from. And through just talking a lot, he said basically that even though we were trying to do our best for him . . . it wasn't us who were going to decide what was going to happen to him, it was Allah. And we talked a lot about that. And once we got to that point where it was out in the open, the pressure was off to try to improve his compliance or adherence or whatever word you want to use. So, every time I see him, we always talk a little bit about spirituality . . . and he asks me to pray for him. . . . And we talk about things like not being able to talk to anybody about his infection because it's not something you discuss openly in a Muslim community, and the fact that there's a lot of pressure being placed on him to get married, but he knew that he couldn't get married because he had an infection, and he wouldn't be able to disclose this to a potential partner. And the expectation is that they would have children. . . . So we had long discussions about this and I don't think that if he'd been seen by a physician that that would have come out. . . . And so I don't pressure him about his medications, and we just kind of understand where we're each coming from.

This story reveals the emergence of what Mishler (1984) referred to as the voice of the patient's lifeworld, which is different from the voice of medicine, which Mishler acknowledged is overwhelmingly characteristic of the medical worldview. In an attempt to provide care, this NP nursed the patient's physical, emotional, and spiritual wounds. Through the creation of a bond with the patient, she tried to diminish the asymmetry in the provider–patient relationship and maximize his input into the encounter. There is no sense of blame or judgment evident in this NP's story or a need to coerce the patient to become compliant with his medication regimen. She does not "medicalize" him. Thus, she avoids closure in each encounter and over time. Instead, she makes herself available and accessible by sharing a piece of herself. The NP lets the patient get to know her, and in doing so, she legitimizes his feelings about his life and illness.

By sharing her own cultural and religious beliefs, this NP identifies herself as both similar to and different from her patient, legitimizing her patient's experiences and opening up the opportunity to reflect on these differences in new ways. She knows her patient as someone whom she affects, and she knows herself as affected by the patient who has become part of who she is as an NP. In doing so, the NP resists dominant cultural assumptions. Mikhail Bakhtin (quoted by Frank 2004, p. 20) calls this *deepest communion*: "To be means to be for another, and through the other." This communion is what makes this moment moral. In being connected through dialogue, the NP and the patient are within a relation in which they hear, recognize, and remember each other. This is the premise underlying Gadow's (1980) proposal that to regard "the patient as a 'whole' would seem to require nothing less than the nurse acting as a whole person. Therefore, the person who withdraws parts of the self is unlikely to allow the patient to emerge as a whole, or to comprehend that wholeness if it does emerge" (p. 87). By being open, receptive, and available, the NP was present to the Other. Gabriel Marcel (1948) put it his way: "The person who is at my disposal is the one who is capable of being with me with the whole of himself when I am in need; while the one who is not at my disposal seems merely to offer me a temporary loan raised on his resources. For the one I am a presence; for the other I am an object" (p. 26).

Connecting with patients by opening oneself also demonstrates that the NP–patient relationship is not built on a foundation of patient incompetence. The patient is treated as the expert on his own life and as such is free to choose his own course. "Committing yourself to dialogue with people is more than recognizing their inherent dignity and defending their rights; it's being willing to allow their voice to count as much as yours" (Frank, 2004, p. 44).

The NP in this story did not independently define what was medically relevant, or simply confine medical relevancy to the patient's medical symptoms; rather, she repeatedly made attempts to create a genuine opportunity for connectedness by generously offering herself in terms of time, space, and person. She left the way open for psychosocial issues to structure the exchange and be part of the meaning of the illness event. By viewing NPs' practice through the family therapy work of nurses Wright, Watson, and Bell (1996), we realize that, for NPs, the goal of being connected is to enable their patients to discover how they want to live and to find the resources to do so. They do not regard diagnostic labelling of the individual as a useful vocabulary with which to work.

It is not uncommon for communication among multiple consulting physicians, various team members, and family members, in addition to the patient, to increase the complexity of decision-making. This can be particularly difficult for NPs who are involved in developing and implementing the medical treatment plan of care but who still do not hold the ultimate authority. However, for NPs, the decision-making process involves being connected.

There was one family in particular that their daughter was quite unwell, and I was giving the results of the ultrasound of the kidneys to this mom and dad. And it was not the results they wanted to hear, but the kidneys just weren't working anymore. And the question being: Was transplant an option? And they said, "If it was your baby, what would you do?" And it was such a hard question for me. Everybody else was: "No, transplant's not an option, can't even think about it." But when they sat and asked me, "What would you do?" it was like, "If it was my kid, honestly," I said, "I don't know. I guess I'd have to just think how much they were suffering. If there was any hope that it would work, they could still be alive and have a life or the life they still had, I would be doing it. It's just two ways of looking at it." . . . It was a very emotional situation. They were very sad. We were all crying. But, they understood where I was coming from. They appreciated that, because they were getting so much of "Just stop now." But it was very clear for me that this family couldn't live with the guilt of not having given her every single option or opportunity, and in this mom's mind she had to look at every opportunity or option, and as a mom I could see the same thing.

In this situation, "Gloria," the NP, does not reproduce the hegemonic medical understanding of the case. She supports the parents and, in doing so, speaks an oppositional discourse. Rather than say as little as possible and retreat into silence, she opens herself to the parents. She reveals herself as human by openly expressing her emotions, acknowledging the parents' suffering by sharing it with them, "demonstrating that she too is human (as in 'fallible')," which fundamentally changes any perceived power imbalance between them (Hawley, 2005, p. 119). Moreover, by not shying away from the mother's question — "If it was your baby, what would you do?" Gloria experiences a microethical moment in her practice; and holding to the difficult, she lets the mother know that she understands her dilemma and the guilt parents may experience. Gloria calls on her own position as a woman and a mother to be as empathetic as possible. Even while they remain provider and "patient" (an extension of the infant), they relate to each other as women and as parents. The sharing of tears was not a crossing of professional boundaries but rather an opening of self. The NP is in the situation with the parents, and for that moment she shares their burden.

Positioning herself in a community of parents, Gloria identifies herself as like the parents. On this basis of solidarity she legitimizes their experiences, their values and beliefs, their feelings, and their choices. She acknowledges that she recognizes them. These dialogues are examples of what Frank (2004) described as a practice of generosity, where forming relationships of connectedness helps to diminish feelings of isolation for both the patient and family, and even the care provider. NPs are able to witness patients' and families' attempts to understand themselves as morally responsible persons. Likewise, in being witnesses connected with others, NPs are able to recognize themselves as morally responsible.

This does not mean that NPs do not struggle with the choices that patients or their families make, particularly those which are self-destructive. They may repeatedly offer the same "medical" recommendations and even show their frustration. However, many NPs reveal that they attempt to avoid closure by neither imposing their medical expertise nor their impression of the definition of the situation. By remaining in a dialogue, NPs keep open the possibility that the patient, and even they, may "interrupt the monological pursuit of their own purposes and self-perceptions" (Frank, 2004, p. 45):

I can get extremely frustrated with a client but at the same time
I still think about where they're coming from, and maybe where

they're coming from isn't necessarily where I'm coming from. . . .
A patient that I have been working with for a number of years —
he has a substance abuse problem — he phoned me and said,
"I won't be in for my appointment tomorrow because I've checked
myself into [drug recovery program]." So after five years of planting
the seed, picking him up, picking up the pieces, having him come
into the clinic drunk, and just being there all the time and never
really judging him in any way, the fact that he called me . . .
I just said to him, "That's wonderful; that's fantastic," and I said,
"When you're finished, you have to come and see me and tell me all
about it." But that's a really good day; that's a really good day.

NPs strive to engage in relationships with their patients and families in a way that is collaborative, reciprocal, negotiated, and
participatory. They do not tell their patients how they should
deal with the problems in their lives; instead, they put forward
some things for them to consider. They explain the importance
of health-related interventions and treatment options, teach their
patients how to care for themselves, make recommendations, and
circle the issues in multiple ways, revisiting them from a variety
of angles. They seek to guide their patients through the illness
event, helping them to find the path that best fits with their personal goals and aspirations. However, they do so in ways that
minimize the distance between themselves and their patients,
such that even when the NPs' treatment recommendations are
not chosen, the connectedness is maintained and the possibilities for further negotiation for care remain open. Helen shared
her attempts to help her patient with a lung tumour better manage her pain, which resulted from a severe cough and radiation
therapy. Although her symptoms were relieved with cough and
pain medications, the patient discontinued their use once her
symptoms dissipated, only to have them reoccur shortly thereafter. Helen acknowledged that the patient was reluctant to take

them because they made her "feel sleepy and spacey," but Helen also observed that if her cough and pain were bad, then she had difficulties coping. Despite her frustration, Helen still thought "about where she's coming from" and used multiple opportunities to help her see the use and management of these medications in a different way:

> I said, "Well you don't have to take anything. . . . However, I do think if you take the injection of the pain-management drug we've ordered before you go for your radiation treatment you'll probably get through it better, because what I'm not sure is if it's just lying on that hard table that's making your back sore. . . . If it's flared up from this treatment then I think we may have our answer, and then the trick is to take something pretty strong before you go over. . . . But you time when you take your pain medication, you time when you take the cough medication, but I might suggest that if it makes you feel dozy during the day then take the bigger dose of cough medicine at bedtime, because you know you don't care if you're dozy at night; you're sleeping right?" And she said, "Yeah, that makes sense to me." Anyway, we're working on that.

Even within the constraints of a busy practice, NPs struggle to give the time and personal attention that helps patients to feel that they are being heard and not rushed. As Mishler (1984), Fisher (1995), and others have argued, physicians all too often dismiss the social or biographical contexts of patients' lives as not the "real stuff" of medicine. By treating the medical and the social as dualities and treating organic pathology as medical, physicians leave the way open for two separate but interrelated phenomena. But what has been revealed here is that many NPs are driven by the ideology to unify the two in their work.

However, not all NPs are able to connect with their patients in this way, nor do all NPs develop these types of relationships with all of their patients, all of the time. As one NP realistically noted, not all patients need or want a close relationship with their care provider. A contrasting example of how NPs may sometimes engage with their patients is offered by "Jamie." She shared her feelings about a patient with known cardiac disease who regularly visited the Emergency Department with chest pain. He had been enrolled in the service's chest program on numerous occasions, but due to a phobia of particular diagnostic tests as a result of a past life event, he failed to make his appointments. "Well, I'm basically fed up with him because every time we go through the same thing. We spend all this time with him trying to explain. I mean, I feel for this man, but I've just been around it so many times. . . . He just doesn't really listen to what I say." Instead of being connected with her patient in a way that helps to unify the psychosocial and biographical context of his life with the medical diagnoses, Jamie separates them. Consequently, there is an underlying sense that she blames the patient for his inability to comply with the treatment plan. As though if he could only control his fears, the proper care could be provided. The patient's inability to take the required diagnostic tests is somehow at odds with the NP's expectations. Because of this, Jamie not only presents the medical system as having definitive authority, but she also prevents any opportunities for the patient to discover new possibilities for healing.

Thus, not all NPs practice in a patient-centred, holistic manner or with a spirit of generosity all of the time, even though it is espoused as their intention and alleged to be highly valued. Many struggle to maintain their commitment to being connected. A few talked about managing their patients and their families, discussing them in terms of cases or diagnoses. They listed the multiple barriers that prevented them from entering into relations of care, and the frustration that they experienced with feeling unconnected. The list included such reasons as the volume of patients to be seen, expedient transfers from one unit to another, the location of offices relative to the practice settings, the actual time spent on-service given the number of NPs within the service, and the other parts of the job that result in less time for being accessible to the patients and families.

The serious question is whether any of the reasons for circumventing connectedness are *good* reasons. Some NPs need to care for the patient right from the time of admission in order to feel connected: "I feel bonded when they are admitted and that's usually when they're the sickest . . . whereas, if you get this patient whom you've never met them before, then you don't have that bond and it's much, much harder." However, some NPs are able to create connectedness despite being off-service, challenging spatiotemporal factors, early transfers, or multiple care providers: "I make a point of meeting with the parents, even the week that I'm off-service, because I feel and want a certain connectedness with them. . . . I say hi, and check on them. . . . And if they have a few questions, I answer those to the best of my knowledge, and then refer them to my colleagues who are on-service for the details."

The role external factors play as barriers to being connected should not be discounted in any way. All NPs are challenged by a variety of situational issues on a daily basis, challenges that hinder engagement with patients and families in meaningful ways. Yet while many NPs are able to be connected despite these challenges, some are unable to be connected because of them. Does this reflect personal choice or the tendency to be drawn into the vortex that is modern technology? Could this struggle reflect medicine's treatment of patients in terms of what Heidegger (1977, p. 16) describes as "an object on call for inspection" and what Foucault (1994, p. 14) refers to as the "medical gaze"; that is, the patient's body is viewed as an object of inquiry and the individual is a case? In a seminal critique of modern technology, Heidegger argued that technology imposes a particular sorting, ordering, commanding, and disposing of nature and man (p. 16). For example, the hospital is not a building (tool) we use; it is not an object at all, but rather a flexible and efficient (or inefficient) cog in the health care system. Likewise, the patients are not persons who use the health care system, but rather are used by it to fill the hospitals, clinics, and doctors' offices (Rashotte, 2005, p. 53) and, thereby, are transformed into objects for inspection, "subordinate to the orderability" (Heidegger, 1977, p. 18) of the system. Likewise, viewed from a Foucauldian perspective, the patient's body is treated in a machine-like fashion with personal identity stripped away as daily routines, surroundings, and clothes are removed and the patient's voice is silenced and medical interventions undertaken (Leder, 1992, p. 121). Does the augmented use of technology that occurs within NPs' practice — combined with their enhanced engagement with medical practitioners who view the human body as a pathological object through which to clarify diagnosis — promote detachment and less meaningful relationships with their patients?

Certainly, several NPs described the seductive power of medical practice and how easy it is to emulate the medical worldview. Perhaps by viewing the instrumental nature of NP practice as an obstacle to be overcome, NPs are challenged to remake themselves and in the process modify their medical milieu. Heidegger argued that we do not have to be prisoners of technology; rather, the saving power of technology is its ability to demand us to think in another way. He called for a reflective kind of questioning and meditative thinking. Engaging in reflective or meditative thought — which many of the NPs stories heretofore have demonstrated — "grants us the possibility of dwelling in the world in a totally different way [and] promises a new ground and foundation upon which we can stand and endure in the world of technology without being imperilled by it" (Heidegger, 1966, p. 55). Reflection as ontology — that is, a critical analysis in which one learns about oneself and one's way of being — enables us to correct and improve our practices for the purpose of shaping a 'good' nursing model of care (Kim, 1999, p. 1206). This involves reflecting on the ways in which we wish to govern ourselves such that the use of power becomes a relational power (Foucault, 1980). Perhaps being committed to being connected both through the use *and* despite the power of modern technology facilitates meaningful NP-patient relationship and is the difference that NPs are able to make in their practice. Being committed to being connected enables NPs practice to arrive at a "medicine of the *intertwining*" (Leder, 1992, p. 125), which involves and promotes "a chiasmatic blending of biological and existential" (p. 125) dimensions of care.

NPs often extend the provision of information, support, and referrals as well as the promotion of coping strategies beyond individual patients to their families and support networks. NPs recognize that the latter also need comfort and information during their loved one's acute illness. NPs strive to create moments with family members to foster connected relationships. For example, the simple acts of stopping to chat, touching base on a daily basis, phoning families who cannot visit to provide them with an update, or staying behind to discuss concerns that are just touched upon in rounds are all examples of being connected.

It's very common during bedside rounds . . . for one of us to stay behind, even if it's not a nurse practitioner's patient, and I say, "Did you understand what he said, or do you have any questions about that?" . . . Even if it's something that is minor to us, well sometimes the parents are just flabbergasted, and I've seen my [NP] colleagues stop and take the time and even put an arm around the mom or something. You never see a physician do that, not even a female physician . . . that's a nursing thing.

NPs demonstrate their connectedness through their ability to be *compassionate*, a word derived from the Latin words *cum* and *patior*, which together mean "to suffer with" (Barnhart, 1988). Leder (1990) indicates that compassion refers to an experiencing-with another, and in the act of sharing another's experience, one is able to recognize the experience of the Other as a possible experience of oneself (van Manen, 1991). Compassion is the NPs' justification for putting their arms around the Other or stepping away from rounds to spend time explaining or answering families' questions and concerns. If one recognizes the power of information to create anxiety, uncertainty, and a further loss of control in the situation, then can it not be perceived as abandonment in the moment to simply throw out information and turn away? Instead, NPs help patients and family members comprehend the information given to them by simplifying and adapting the medical language, thus empowering them to become partners in care. Although using medical jargon and the medical mode of speaking with physicians in front of families fosters the families' confidence in NPs as caregivers, when NPs translate that same information with an intentionality of respect and partnership, the interconnectedness between the NP and the family is deepened and strengthened. These acts represent the ways in which NPs strive to draw the families into a relation of care; "because care can only be a relationship, a dialogue not only of words but of touch" (Frank, 2004, p. 27), either literal or metaphorical.

The clinical practice in the acute-care setting involves communication and coordination with multiple specialty physicians, various institutional services, and outside community agencies. A large part of NPs' practices involves being connected with the patient and family across and through time and place through a process of coordinating this complex system. NPs create constancy, consistency, and continuity, with the intent to ease the burden that being within the health care system tends to cause, and to ensure that patients and families do not fall through the cracks. They do what Hawley (2005) has referred to as making the inhumane humane. The experience of being in this system is one of dehumanization (Gadow, 1980; Foucault, 1994) — invasion of privacy, infringement of autonomy, being viewed as object and rendered invisible — and it is real and ever-present in health care as it is currently structured.

"Joan," (who was introduced in an earlier section) was concerned for those groups of individuals who did not know how to negotiate the health care system, such as newly immigrated families, those with poor language skills, those living in and out of the correctional system, those with mental health issues, or people otherwise living with somewhat chaotic lives and with limited resources. Joan believed that all of these individuals needed someone to support them, provide them with education about their illness, assist them with illness-related problems or treatments, help them negotiate multiple care providers, and provide health promotion, such as dealing with smoking cessation, cardiovascular health, and substance abuse. She felt that these needs arise largely because physicians who are very specialized in their knowledge do not deal with these issues in their practice. As well, these patients either tend not to have a family physician, or the family physician refuses to see them once they repeatedly fail to show for appointments.

Joan recognized the chaotic nature of these patients' lives, lives that do not necessarily fit into a time structure or appreciate the importance of showing up on time for prescheduled appointments. Thus she created a "one-stop-care" practice. Although she arranged appointments with them, if they did not show up, were an hour late, or decided to come at four o'clock on Friday though they were expected at nine o'clock, she would still welcome and see them. As a result, more and more of these patients called her directly because they saw her as their primary-care provider.

Eventually family physicians and other nurses in the community of public health recognized that she could see somebody quickly. She did not work in isolation but negotiated this philosophy of practice with the other members of the team. Eventually they were willing for her to create this alternative form of time embedded within the traditional time structure of appointments: "Everybody knows that I could be with somebody for a half hour or I could be there for two hours," and "when people come at weird times when I'm not expecting them to show up, basically what I do is I put things on hold and just say, Okay, this is the most important thing to do right now, and so I spend time with the patient."

Being connected through constancy, consistency, and continuity involves worrying about the Other and then acting upon that worry. NPs work the system through such actions as massaging egos, calling in favours, crossing professional boundaries, and negotiating with one's colleagues for the chance to create time and space in order to better care for Others. Being connected is recognizing that care has to happen within a relationship, which is different for each patient and family. One NP commented that for many patients and families, the "relationship is a professional one, in which they don't know much about you and you don't know much about them, and that's okay, and the care is outside of their own sense of well-being." But for some, the care "happens inside a specific relationship, and, if it doesn't happen inside that relationship, it isn't going to happen." NPs encourage the patients and their families to define the relationship across time and place, as long as it isn't outside the boundaries of NP practice. Consistency and continuity within their practice allows for caring moment to moment. Opportunities are enhanced to know individuals more fully as human beings with hopes, dreams, and aspirations, and for using every creative, imaginative, and innovative way possible to help them to live more fully and to grow as human beings.

Being Content

Both the world and beyond the world, free as a bird, the
self searches for a third space, singing, dancing, nesting,
and flying, sometimes with companions, sometimes alone,
always already attending to the call of the stranger.
(Wang, 2004, p. 138)

As an adjective, the word *content*, derived from the Latin word *con-tentus*, means to be satisfied, pleased, gratified, and even delighted.
Being content with being an NP means experiencing a sense of
satisfaction, and even joy, with what the NP does in his or her
clinical practice. The word *content* also implies the sum of the
constituent elements of something, such as the totality of the
constituents of a person's experience at any particular moment.
The NPs' experience of satisfaction is the sum of the constituent
elements of being competent, confident, comfortable, committed, and connected, recognizing that the sum of the elements
as co-experienced and interrelated is, as a whole, more than
and different from the parts. Finally, the word *conten*, means the
allaying of doubt and the satisfying of the conscience. In being
confident with their competence, and comfortable that they are
able to embody their practice in a way that demonstrates being
committed and connected, NPs find that their doubts about what
they do and how they do it are allayed, such that they experience a strong sense of doing what is both right and good. Being
content is about finding a fit in being an NP.

NPs want to do something manifestly practical in the clinical
setting: stay close to the patients and their families. They find
this in the direct clinical practice component of the NP role. "It's
about diagnosing and coming up with the solution," about "the

actual doing of the procedure," and "the sense of success when you have the line in the right place." "It's being able to complete the plan, the intervention, and then the re-evaluation of it, and being satisfied at the end of it that the patient is in the best outcome that can possibly be." They no longer feel constrained. They have ample independence, autonomy, and added responsibility and accountability. They are able to work collaboratively and build partnerships with their medical colleagues, in a way that feels safe. They are able to be involved in every aspect of the patients' and families' care by developing relationships with them over time. They are continually challenged, recognized, and valued for what they do. In other words, they discover a niche in nursing. They are glad they have made the journey and believe they have made the right choice. They are happy with how it turned out and have no regrets. Being an NP suits them and they feel satisfied. Being content affects the dialogical engagement with self and Others and consequently they renegotiate how they understand who they are as NPs in their practice.

NPs recognize that some of their NP colleagues are entranced by the medical realm and seem to leave their nursing values behind, which potentially leaves the patient vulnerable. One NP observed, "That's the danger of this role . . . opportunity and danger coexist on the same line." NPs admit how easy it is to be "seduced by the dark side," which does not mean medicine is "the bad side," but that there is a great deal of power associated with prescriptive authority and the language associated with ordering. One NP noted, "You can choose to keep that [power] to yourself or you can choose to share it. It is a struggle and sometimes it's just easier to be on the medical side." For some NPs, being content only concerns the attainment of more autonomy, control, recognition, and power. To be seen as the captain of the ship, or at least a welcome sailor, is the desired fit. Being totally aligned with physicians is perceived as a reasonable means to a desirable end, allowing NPs to "accomplish plans with others through access to traditional power sources" (Rafael, 1996, p. 13).

For many NPs, the natural state of complexity inherent in the process of being and becoming an NP exposes the contradictions in the experience of their practice, yet it also provides the opportunity to reconcile these contradictions. For example, many nurses drawn to the NP role have seen nurses working at the bedside as invisible, not valued, and "impotent in effecting the social and political changes necessary to transform their clients' realities" (Rafael, 1996, p. 6). To acquire power, some NPs may distance themselves from other nurses by valuing knowledge and skills from other disciplines over nursing knowledge, or totally aligning themselves with medicine. Power, in what Rafael has called assimilated caring (p. 8), is acquired by aligning with medical characteristics, practice, and behaviours and by integrating medical norms. An NP who speaks with disdain about the physicians' inability to see the patients "crumpled up at the bottom of the bed" while on rounds but subsequently "gets the nurse to reposition the patients so they're more comfortable while we're busy talking about their plan of care for the day" provides an example of distancing from nursing. NPs who echo the dominant medical discourse — which is that nurses' key skills are those associated primarily with information gathering and the means by which they carry out medical orders — also exhibit this form of distancing. One NP said, "Nurses just usually follow orders. They're there to gather the data that's needed. It's vital to have that information, but we're the ones who put it together and try to find the solution." Another observed, "There are a wide variety of nurses in the field and how they think, but many of them don't think; they just do what the procedures are and they are not thinking about why they're doing it."

However, the cost of power obtained in this way may cause professional disunity, a lowering of professional self-esteem, and a feeling of being marginalized. In fact, nurses' caring remains devalued, thus fostering a lived contradiction. In addition, Bates (1990, p. 139) — a physician, the author of the classic physical examination text, and a strong proponent of the NP role — warned that "by expanding into medicine, nurse practitioners will need more than ever before to increase their consciousness of what nursing is all about. The values of nursing must not get lost in the dominant medical cultures. If they do, nurse practitioners justly risk the epithet of *junior doctor*."

Many NPs resist the dominant discourse that associates medicine with independence, cognitive logic, and aggression, and nursing with dependence, nurturing, and emotive logic (Rafael, 1996, p. 3). These characteristics are no longer viewed as conflicting concepts or as superior and inferior ways of knowing and being. Instead, NPs demonstrate in their actions the power that comes from diversity, voice, nurturance, responsibility, knowledge sharing, and choice, deeply intertwined with autonomy, strength, mastery, and assertiveness. No one denies that traditional power *over* may be used as a means to an end, such as to influence action in a health care system that is in need of change. However, a strong emphasis on mutual power exists, such that NP, patient, and other care providers are transformed during the relationship, balancing out the power *between*. NPs who argue that the question should always be: *What do the patients need?* — and not *What do the docs need?* or *What do the nurses need?* — exemplify the move from *power* as being embedded in a division of labour that primarily serves the interests of those in power, to *power* as enabling, with opportunities for being equal in relations. Power as enabling is a relational way of being and becoming for these NPs. It is demonstrated in their heightened awareness of interrelatedness. It emerges as a sense of responsibility and generosity toward Others, in a practice informed by various forms of knowledge and skill, and it presupposes a growing knowledge base and clinical competence. For these NPs, being content means practising within this ontological, epistemological, and ethical understanding of power in praxis.

NPs are frequently asked by patients, nurses, physicians, and their own friends and families if they feel more like a nurse or more like a physician in the administration of their practice. Do they live in the medical world or that of nursing? As they become competent, confident, and comfortable with the knowledge and skills required in the performance of their practice, embedded within being committed and connected, NPs begin to experience an inner transformation. They no longer resist the tasks traditionally associated with the medical world, nor do they dread the questions *Who are you?* and *Where is your allegiance?* They have endured the tumultuous seas of being adrift and overcome their fears by facing the most frightening places within themselves. Now, a new way of being in nursing is discovered within each encounter in the practice setting, and they discover all or part of the new dream or vision for their professional practice.

I'm a nurse. I think building those core relationships with the nursing staff and making sure you are aligned with nursing is important. And it's very easy to slip into the physician's world, to align too closely with the physicians. And the physicians will say, "You're as good as a doctor," and they mean that as a compliment, but I say, "Always remember I'm a nurse. I do not want to be seen as a mini-doctor." But, I also mean that I'm part of the physician team too. And so, hopefully, I am the best of nursing and the best of medicine and I'm just broader, or rounder, but different. Is it a third mindset maybe? But it's not necessarily separate, more of a joined mindset.

Amin Maalouf (2000), who was born and raised in Lebanon but lived and worked for 22 years in France, wrote that he always gave the same answer to the question of whether he is more French or more Lebanese: "Both." He explained, "What makes me myself rather than anyone else is the very fact that I am poised between two countries, two or three languages and several cultural traditions. It is precisely this that defines my identity" (p. 1). "Would I exist more authentically if I cut off a part of myself?" he asked. Similarly, would NPs exist more authentically if they cut off a part of themselves? Are NPs half-nurse and half-physician? Of course not. And despite the vast difference between identity considered in terms of ethnic origins and identity considered in terms of professional roles, identity in both cases cannot be compartmentalized. As Maalouf (p. 2) wrote, "You can't divide it up into halves or thirds or any other separate segments."

After giving a detailed account of why he lays claim to all his affiliations, Maalouf observed that someone always seeks to know what he truly feels "deep down inside." This question seems to reflect the widespread view that deep down inside there is just one affiliation that really matters, a kind of fundamental truth about each individual, an essence determined once and for all when one belongs to a group or discipline. It is as "if the rest, all the rest — a person's whole journey through time as a free agent; the beliefs he acquires in the course of that journey; his own individual tastes, sensibilities and affinities; in short, his life itself — counted for nothing" (Maalouf, 2000, p. 2). When NPs are asked who they are and where they belong, they are meant to seek within themselves such an alleged fundamental allegiance. Having located it, they are then supposed to flaunt it proudly in the face of others. Is this not what the current debate about the role of the NP is about? Does the current discourse expounding the lack of allegiance to nursing through their engagement in "physician tasks" not marginalize NPs for claiming a more complex identity?

NPs follow a quasi-Hegelian dialectical journey as they engage in the doing of clinical practice, during which internal contradictions are transcended but give rise to new contradictions that require resolution. Thus, the journey shifts back and forth between an ongoing unmaking and remaking, shaping each NP's particular experience. Frank (2004) observes, "Doing is what counts, and knowing what counts as worth doing depends on being a person who has become shaped through discipline" (p. 53). NPs continue to define who they are by where they have been in nursing as well as where they are going in their current role. By doing within a community of practice, NPs experience a change in their behaviour and performance. They know themselves no longer as people who only perform the tasks of taking histories, doing physicals, diagnosing, or prescribing, but as people who bring comfort to patients and families, always recognizing them as persons with whom their care is entrusted and with whom they are in partnership. They experience a new sense of belonging, and a sense of self is rediscovered in the act of experiencing their practice in a fuller way. In the words of Katerina Clark and Michael Holquist (quoted in Frank 2004, p. 46):

The way in which I create myself is by means of a quest: I go out to the other in order to come back with a self. I "live into" an other's consciousness; I see the world through that other's eyes. But I must never completely meld with that version of things, for the more successfully I do, the more I will fall prey to the limitation of the other's horizon. A complete fusion . . . even if it were possible, would preclude the difference required by dialogue.

Over time, NPs are able to decide which judgments they choose to hold on to and which they will consider not conducive to becoming who they want to be (Frank, 2004, p. 53). New knowledge of self is revealed in the act of practising, and as result they no longer have to address questions about whether they are nurses or physician replacements, or whether their focus is care or cure from a dichotomous position.

In the 2003 book *Aidan's Way: The Story of a Boy's Life and a Father's Journey*, the author, Sam Crane, a professor of Asian studies, wrote of his struggles with his son's rare birth defects and his transformation into the "Father of Disabled Child, a different status, [a role] that was harder to anticipate and freighted with dread and alienation" (p. 51). In "struggling to stay afloat, drifting at the mercy of the deluge" (p. 45), he found himself looking for answers and support in such ancient Chinese texts as the *Book of Changes* and *Tao Te Ching* "in search of a different, perhaps more positive, perspective" (p. 66) on how to live this new life. Frank (2004, p. 31) referred to this turn toward these passages as a way "to make a figurative raft" (p. 31). Through a dialectic engagement with passages from these texts, Crane (2003) grew in his understanding of how to live this new life by seeing his situation in a new way:

> Water yields to its surroundings; it takes the shape and follows the course of the path it finds. Its adaptability gives it a certain resilience, its constancy a certain power — and it maintains these characteristics however precipitous its passage. . . .
>
> The passage did not detail precisely how to adapt to danger, like the stream in the abyss, but it gave me a mental image of how to meet the challenge: take on the shape of the surroundings, fill up the spaces encountered, flow over and around the rocks and falls. (p. 54)

In much the same way, each experience of making a difference engages the NP in a personal dialectic, and those experiences serve as a raft on their journey. Each experience of making a difference in their ordinary, day-to-day practice adds resonance to their personal journey, connecting their struggles and discoveries to an understanding of how to live as NPs, how to understand who they are, and provides a measure of what counts as valuable and meaningful to them as NPs. These experiences, called upon in a dialectic engagement, have their "fulfilment not in definitive knowledge but in the openness to experience that is made possible by experience itself" (Gadamer, 1989, p. 355) and suggest which ways of understanding and acting they should cultivate and which they should avoid in their practice. Experience, from a Gadamerian perspective, is not concerned with the fact that someone already knows everything in the sense of information; rather, "the experienced person proves to be . . . someone . . . who, because of the many experiences he has had and the knowledge he has drawn from them, is particularly well equipped to have new experiences and to learn from them" (p. 355). In other words, experience relates to the emergence of insights that arise from the "many disappointments of one's expectations" (Gadamer, 1989, p. 356) and the learning that occurs through suffering (p. 356). As a result of this type of experience, the values that NPs uphold become self-disclosed as well as evident to others. By using their new knowledge and skills competently, confidently, and comfortably, they affect their own representation of who they are as NPs through the way they do their work and relate to others. They reveal the moral framework within which they choose to live.

Being content means NPs realize that being an NP does not require them to abandon a nursing framework of care. NPs' stories are replete with moments of both care and cure, as well as their performance in both the nursing and medical domains. The medical domain contains diagnosis and treatment of diseases. The nursing domain contains consideration of individual and family responses to actual or potential threats to health and involves helping patients cope with disease processes that might be occurring. NPs anticipate human distress and work on the level of what an illness experience means to the patient and family. They bring together two traditions of thought that are intrinsic not only to the process of negotiating how to care for their patients, but also to the meaning of who they are as NPs. The complementarity of nursing and medicine reflects the fundamental inherent duality of who NPs are and what they do in clinical practice. This duality is a fundamental aspect of the identity of being an NP. Simply stated, medicine and nursing are two interacting dimensions embodied by the NP; they do not define a spectrum, for to regard them in this way is to still see a relationship between opposites, where "moving to one side implies leaving the other. More of one implies less of the other" (Wenger, 1998, pp. 66–67). As Wenger (1998) illustrated, with an interacting duality, both elements are always involved, and both can take different forms and degrees. In fact, the NPs' practice can be construed as stemming from their ability to bring the two together.

This does not mean, however, that NPs want to, in Maalouf's (2000, p. 21) terms, "dissolve" their identities "in a kind of undifferentiated and colourless soup." Increasing the level of involvement in medicine or nursing does not dispense with the other. On the contrary, it will tend to increase and transform the requirement of the other. Wenger (1998, p. 68) posited that a binary or dichotomy "tends to suggest that there must be a process by which one can move from one to the other by translation into a different but equivalent state." For example, when NPs prescribe, either their actions are ascribed to those of a physician substitute (and subsequently their identities would be translated as thus), or the prescriptive act is interpreted merely as a tool in the nurse's hands, passed on by medicine. By contrast, a change in the relationship between nursing and medicine within a single role always transforms the possibilities for negotiating meaning. Participating in the medical world is not just a functional enactment of a set of prescribed tasks, but a renegotiation of what it means to be a nurse in this new context. In fact, engagement in these medical activities creates the conditions for new meanings. Perhaps being an NP is like being in a frontier zone criss-crossed by knowledge, skills, language, and geography. But by virtue of this situation — peculiar rather than privileged — NPs have a special role to play in forging links, eliminating misunderstandings, smoothing out difficulties, seeking compromise. Being an NP means having the ability to act as a bridge, a mediator among the various communities and cultures.

And they say, "Are you more like a doctor or are you more like a nurse? And I say, "Well I'd say kind of somewhere in between." But I'm still a nurse. I see a gap, I bridge it. So, sometimes I feel like a bridge builder.

Ted Aoki, a prominent Japanese-Canadian avant-garde pedagogical scholar, entreats us to stop and reflect on what it means to dwell in-between two worlds. In his essay, *Imaginaries of "East and West": Slippery Curricular Signifiers in Education*, Aoki (2005) recalls the time he served as a university representative on a committee engaged in revising a humanities program and the discussion that ensued regarding the entitling of a course, which focused on enlarging students' vision of the world. Suggestions such as "Western and non-Western Civilizations" or "Eastern and non-Eastern Civilizations" were generated; "Western and Eastern Civilizations" was the compromise. It was as a result of this experience that Aoki began a journey of philosophical reflection on the binary image of the terms "East" and "West" as compared to the term "East and West." As Aoki (2005, p. 315) reflected: "The labels 'East' and 'West' suggest two distinct cultural wholes, 'Eastern culture' and 'Western culture,' each identifiable standing distinctly separate from each other" whereas "the term 'East and West' is rendered as a binary of two separate pre-existing entities, which can be bridged or brought together to conjoin in an 'and.'" Furthering his reflections he played with the words bridge and bridging, appreciating the meaning of the words both as a link that enhances movement between places with greater efficiency and a structure that entices a person to linger and dwell, a place where "we are in no hurry to cross over" (Aoki, 2005, p. 317), such as those encountered in Oriental gardens.

Bringing Aoki's reflections into play, we can place quotation marks around "nurse" and "physician" to remind us that both terms are rendered as a binary of two separate pro-existing entities. We can bridge these identities with an "and" when we think of "nurse/nursing and physician/medicine." For an NP, "being a bridge / bridging" could be seen as acting in ways that expedite service, helping patients to move from one place to another in a speedier fashion, thus retaining an instrumental form of being. Such a perspective has implications for nursing, medicine, and administration at a variety of levels. An excessive emphasis on the formalization of the medical world (i.e., the knowledge, skill, and authorization) without corresponding levels of formalized acknowledgment of the nursing expression of the role would, in fact, result in an experience of meaninglessness for NPs. Conversely, a neglect of explanations and formal structures necessary to enable enactment of the medical components of the role would also result in this same experience.

For NPs, clinically managing patients always rests on participating in the medical world: what is said, represented, or otherwise brought into focus in clinical practice must now always assume a history of participation as a context for the interpretation of how they are seen by others, how they see themselves, and how they enact their role. In turn, how they enact the role and how their identity is shaped are always organized around nursing because they come to the role deeply rooted in their nursing history, in the artifacts, language, and concepts that shape nurses' values and beliefs.

Thus, for NPs, nursing is not freed from medicine; in terms of meaningfulness in becoming and being an NP, the opposite is more likely. To be understood and to understand themselves meaningfully, NPs must maintain a close connection to the medical community while not obviating the enactment of the role from a nursing perspective. NPs who have been obstructed from participating in the medical world — that is, they are prevented from enacting the medical components of their role, such as prescribing or performing medical skills they have been trained and licensed to do, or have been asked to step aside when residents are available — find less meaning to their role, not more. Similarly, when they are unable to assimilate their nursing world into the medical one, as when they are adrift, they also experience less meaning to their role. Rather, as Aoki (2005, p. 316) wrote, we may view bridge/bridging in a Heideggerian sense, as "a site or clearing in which earth, sky, mortals and divine in their longing to be together belong together." From this viewpoint, being an NP means that the bridge between nurse and physician is a dwelling place for NPs.

Dwelling on the bridge
In exile between kingdoms
With the stars at night

– Mika Yoshimoto (2008, p. xi)

And I'm always between nursing and medicine, always, always, always. But it's not always a conflictual thing. . . . It is the place where I live. I am a nurse, yet I've got this medical training. I order tests, I read tests. That's not a nursing task. Yet I do some of the parent comforting, I do some of the nursing teaching. So, I'm

*always in between and it's most often not an uncomfortable place.
It's an okay place to be. And sometimes you don't feel you belong,
but sometimes you do. . . . Where do I want to belong? I'd like
to belong to both I guess. I like my attachment to nursing. I like
the way nursing looks at patient care. I like the way nursing is
holistic. Nursing is who I am. . . . I also feel that I have a privileged
relationship with my attending physician and the fellows. Do I
belong in either group fully? I don't think so. But that's okay.*

When NPs state that they feel like they are "neither," or "both,"
or "in no man's land," and even for those who have found their
existential place of being in nursing with the use of medicine,
perhaps they are trying to articulate something akin to Aoki's
image of "crossing" between "East" and "West." Aoki (2005) wrote
that to loosen his attachment to East or West as "thing," he called
upon the Chinese character that "reads 'nothing' or 'no-thing'.":

> But I note that in "no-thing" there is already inscribed the
> word "thing," as if to say "'nothing' cannot be without
> 'thing'," and "'thing' cannot be without 'no thing'." For me,
> such a reading is already a move away from the modern-
> ist binary discourse of "this and that," or that imaginary
> grounded in an essence called "thing." And now I am drawn
> into the fold of a discursive imaginary that can entertain
> "both this and that," "neither this nor that" — a space of
> paradox, ambiguity and ambivalence. (p. 317)

If being an NP is reframed as belonging to both nursing and
medicine, or to neither nursing nor medicine, and if "and" is
re-understood as Aoki's "both 'and' and 'not-and', that allows a
space for both conjunction and disjunction" (Aoki 2005, p. 318),
with bridges being both bridges and non-bridges. NPs' ontological being can be rethought of as a third space between nursing

and medicine. Perhaps this is a new way to consider the meaning of the terms *no man's land*, *my own world*, or *the middle ground* to which some NPs refer. And then, as suggested by Aoki, "identity" is "'identification,' a becoming in the space of difference," "a generative space of possibilities, a space wherein in tensioned ambiguity newness emerges" (Aoki, 2005, p. 318).

Stuart Hall (1990, p. 223) wrote, "Cultural identities come from somewhere, have histories. . . . Far from being eternally fixed to some essentialized past, they are subject to the continuous play of histories, culture, and power." Similarly Maalouf (2000, p. 13) observed that "while there is always a certain hierarchy among the elements that go to make up individual identities this hierarchy is not immutable; it changes over time, and in so doing brings about fundamental changes in behaviour." In this light, NPs are viewed in a space of being content with being in their role, because within this space they share linguistic, geographical, and other cultural elements of both the nursing and medical worlds — "a hybrid of both individual identity and doubled identity" (Aoki, 2005, p. 318) — is created. Brykczynski (1985, p. 5) wrote that the NP is the true hybridization of nursing and medicine. And Ernesto Laclau (1995, quoted in Aoki, 2005, p. 319) noted, "Hybridization does not necessarily mean decline through a loss of identity; it can also mean empowering existing identities through the opening of new possibilities. Only a conservative identity, closed on itself, could experience hybridization as a loss." Indeed, Aoki's imagery allows envisaging of this meaning of a bridge as a third space between worlds. Similarly we can conceive of medicine and nursing as worlds to be bridged, between and among diverse segments of nursing, as spaces of generative possibilities, spaces where newness can flow.

Being an NP can be understood to mean building bridges between one discipline and another, between one part of the health care system and another, taking an active part on both sides, and having an identity that is simultaneously "both" and "not-both." This perspective demonstrates precisely why the unification of dualities is so significant, and possibly why NPs should not be pressed to take sides or ordered to stay totally within their own discipline. Anne Fadiman (1997) in her book *The Spirit Catches You and You Fall Down*, reflects these thoughts most eloquently:

> I have always felt that the action most worth watching is not at the center of things but where edges meet. I like shorelines, weather fronts, international borders. There are interesting frictions and incongruities in these places, and often, if you stand at the point of tangency, you can see both sides better than if you were in the middle of either one. This is especially true, I think, when the apposition is cultural. (viii)

An example from the NPs' world brings to life the reality of being a bridge as an in-between or third space that creates new possibilities:

> Nurses still perceive me as one of them. There are many situations in this unit where nursing and medicine see things differently. . . . Nurses tend to want to move more quickly towards palliative care or comfort care, and we'll question more frequently why we keep going; and for medicine, as long as we haven't exhausted all the avenues, then we're not done. So I'm a bit between and that's very demanding psychologically too. . . . So, for example, a very frequent issue is comfort. Nurses are very pro-comfort. Physicians are pro-comfort as long as they don't want to extubate. . . . And physicians will say, "Well, turn off all the sedation and let the kid wake up," and the nurses are the ones literally sitting on the kid and seeing this child cry and being uncomfortable. And sometimes they see me a bit as a traitor because I'm the one who actually writes the order — stop,

d/c sedation. . . . So I'm seen a bit as a traitor by the nursing team, but sometimes the medical team sees me a bit as a traitor too, as "Stop being a nurse now." . . . But I can see that both parties need to be defended. So I go to my attending and I say, "Well, I don't think we should stop sedation because this kid's been on it for so many days," and I try to negotiate. Usually I get part of what I want at least, and when I come back to the nurses I say, "Well, okay, we got them to halve the sedation rather than stop it." And there's times where it's, "Stop the sedation," and I can understand what the medical rationale is . . . and that comfort is not an issue at this point in time, and that we have to move on. And I think trying to explain to the bedside nurse why and to also say, "Well, if we get into trouble, I'll be there and I'll try to find a solution for you." I think that my role with nursing, it's trying to see if we can find another solution, and with medicine, it's trying to negotiate.

Being an NP is an enriching and fertile experience when NPs feel free to live fully, when they are encouraged to accept their clinical practice in all of its diversity. But it can be hurtful if they are met with looks or words of incomprehension, mistrust, and even outright hostility whenever they claim to be nurses, or if every time they emphasize their ties to the medical world other nurses look on them as traitors or renegades. "[W]ho we are is produced by the effects of our movements among layers of differences" (Pinar and Irwin, 2005, p. 24). That is, the NP's identity it is a negotiated experience, a nexus of multiple memberships, and a relationship between the local and the global (Wenger, 1998, p. 149): others' attitudes must allow for multiplicity to foster NPs' acceptance of this composite identity with tranquillity.

Being content does not mean that the journey comes to an end, even for those NPs who have found the perfect fit. One only has to recall Homer's Odysseus on the Isle of Circe to be reminded that a journey continues because the call for more beckons, there is an external pull to pursue the search for more. After Odysseus had spent many years of bitter wanderings and woes suffered upon the seas, Circe urged him to stay on her island to rediscover the man he had been before he left Ithaca. He stayed with her for well over a year, forgetting to mark the passage of time, content with the fine food and honey-sweet wine, spellbinding songs, and enchanting women, until one day his men came to him to remind him that Ithaca called and that they needed to return to their homes. Then he, too, remembered his people and his obligation, and began to look for the opportunity to continue his journey.

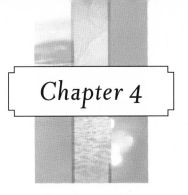

Chapter 4

Being Pulled to Be More

Wenger (1998) argued that the work of identity — in other words, being and becoming — is always ongoing, not in the sense of a fixed course or destination but a continuous motion "that has a momentum of its own in addition to a field of influences" (p. 154). NPs have become who they are — that is, *Being a Nurse Practitioner* — by learning certain ways of playing a part in action with the healthcare team that constitutes their community of practice in the clinical arena. They competently engage in the joint enterprise of caring for a select group of patients in the acute-care setting and participate in a shared repertoire of routines, languages, and genres within this community. But, being an NP is more complex than has been revealed thus far. As is our nature as human beings, the work of identity is always ongoing because it is constructed in multiple social contexts. Furthermore, "identities are defined with respect to the interaction of multiple convergent and divergent trajectories" (Wenger, 1998, p. 154). Finding the perfect fit is one such trajectory, and the dream of what that fit could be provides the context within which NPs determine what learning and activities actually become significant within their role. This sense of trajectory, albeit a course that is not charted or even foreseen in all its variations and permutations, gives them a way of sorting out what matters most, what contributes to their being (and thus their identity), and what remains marginal. NPs are always simultaneously dealing with specific situations, participating in the histories of certain practices, and involved in becoming particular persons. Their journey incorporates their past and their future in the very process of negotiating their present. It is influenced by that which they wish to be and that which others want them to be. Sometimes there is congruence and at other times tension or conflict, but in either case they experience both internal and external struggles. Never is this struggle more evident than in the process of being pulled to be more.

The first and only priority for NPs when they start their journey is necessarily the clinical management of their patients. Keeping their focus entirely on "learning all [they] need to know in the clinical area and to become comfortable doing clinical" is a lengthy process. One NP in her fourth year of clinical practice expressed mixed feelings about her level of clinical expertise and her ongoing development as an NP. She described herself as barely at the point where she could engage in the reflective process of what it meant to be an NP and what had shaped her development. She said, "It's not any one thing, just everything, and nothing" that influenced who she felt she was at this point as an NP, for the entire first two to three years were a blur, the time she was struggling to develop competence, confidence, and comfort with the clinical component of her role. Depending on the nature of their practice — the complexity and variability of patient care, years of experience with the patient population prior to becoming an NP, and relationship with the physician group — it is not unusual for NPs to have been three to five years into their role before they experience and admit to the routine, sometimes even mundane, nature of the direct clinical care they provide and begin to contemplate that they could do more within their practice.

> You spend the first year trying to keep your head above water, trying not to kill anyone, and trying just to get comfortable. And to even suggest you could do education or research the first year is ludicrous in my opinion. The second year you kind of hone and refine your skills, and not just physical skills, but just your whole diagnostic reasoning skills. So you're comfortable on call now by yourself . . . And then, it's not until the third year that you can look outside of yourself for these defining moments because they actually can impact on you then. You can't even take it in before then, really. And I think that that's the point, too, where you have so much more to give and you're ready to take on more in the role and you're ready to mature. . . . So I'm just barely there; I'm just to the point where I can consider and maybe even do more.

Thus as NPs become more efficient and effective in the clinical management of their patients, time and energy become available for them to take on more and different responsibilities in their role. As one NP noted, "when managing patient care begins to run like a well-oiled machine, there is more time to be involved in committee work, education, and research." But, like the initial call to be more, being pulled to be more arises from a variety of internal and external callings.

"They began to give me administrative roles initially," said one NP. "Mostly, it was committee work that I had. I think, after about four years, they gave me responsibility for doing policies and procedures. And now I'm expected to do some element of staff education." For some NPs, the pull arises externally. They find themselves being told about or given added responsibilities by nursing management. Despite acknowledging that the NP role has been set up to include "a clinical portion and to be responsible for some education, some administration, and a small expectation for research," life as an NP is experienced as being only so big, and many feel that they "can't fit it all in." For these NPs, engagement in other advanced nursing practice competencies transpires because of nursing management expectations: "Given that NP salaries are being paid from the nursing budget, NPs need to do things other than just the patient care and contribute back to nursing within the organization or to the program." The concept of "owing the system" is embedded within this perception. However, for NPs who have already found the perfect fit in direct clinical practice, being pulled to be more is experienced as an irritant to be managed and contained, because these extra role functions interfere with the hands-on clinical work they love. As a consequence of "trying to fit in the other parts of the job," noted one NP, there is "less hanging around time" in the unit to be available to meet with families.

> There's always this struggle. Most of the people who stay in this role, I think their primary interest is in patient management, and so if you try and get us too far away from that we're not going to be very happy. How much time do you spend doing this and how much time do you spend doing that? Well, of course, your patient needs are paramount because you can't just leave them be, so they probably take more of your time than what some of the managers would want; but from my point of view, I kind of like that because that's why you're here. You like to do the extra things on the side, but, then they [nursing management] say, "Well, we have this many people so this is how your role is going to be."

Wenger (1998, p. 75) argued that work that is less visible than the more instrumental aspects of practice can easily be undervalued and even totally unrecognized. As a result, some NPs struggle to become engaged in activities that, although desired by some within the more global institutional nursing community, are judged to be of less value by the local community of practice, and by themselves. In fact, for these NPs, being pushed or decreed to produce research or publish more violates their personal definition of a nurse practitioner. Concerned that the organization or nursing administration wants to make "a specialist" out of them, they perceive research, education, and leadership responsibilities to be domains of practice that belong to the CNS role.

As a result of the constant tension experienced between clinical practice and other advanced nursing practice responsibilities, resentment toward management surfaces, and NPs' frustration at not being understood builds. Nursing management comes to be perceived as "they," with power over NPs' time management and energy focus: "If administration is putting out a lot of dollars into some position, then they want to see more nursing output and see that work highlighted throughout the world. It isn't enough to give good patient care; you have to be publishing it." Fear of replacement arises and is compounded by the perception that the physicians with whom they work have little power to intervene on their behalf. They are aware of the discourse about "foreign graduates who can't get on as physicians but who could become physician assistants," and the consequent negative impact this could have on the NP group if they do not meet the service component of the role.

The operating officer of this hospital believes in nurse practitioners, but not strictly as a patient management role, because then that could be seen as physician's assistants or something like that. Somehow this has to be uniquely nursing, and I can buy that. But then what is the split? . . . So our manager is saying, "I think that you spend too much time on the patient management and I want to make sure that you have time for these other roles to make it whatever." But I'm just thinking, Well, make sure that you meet the program needs, because if you don't then they will get physician's assistants and then we'll be unnecessary, and that's not a good thing for us. . . . You can't work that way. If you want the job and you say that you can provide this type of care and yet at the drop of the hat you just let everything go, can you see where people might perceive you as not that important? Like if you're not there to provide the service then somebody else could do it because obviously you're letting them do it.

A strong historical foundation for some NPs' fear of replacement by other professionals undeniably exists. Memories are not so short as to forget that the first NP initiative ended in Ontario, just over 25 years ago, with the closing of the last primary health care NP education program at McMaster University. This occurred because of a perceived oversupply of physicians, lack of a remuneration mechanism, lack of public awareness regarding the NP role, and lack of support for the role from medicine and nursing (Nurse Practitioners Association of Ontario, 2005). Hundreds of newly trained NPs found themselves unemployed as a surplus of new medical graduates flooded the market. NPs, seen merely as physician replacements, were no longer needed or wanted. It is also a fact that some legitimately qualified NPs have replaced nurses who had been permitted to engage in advanced roles without adequate qualifications, and who subsequently lost their jobs. Many nurses seized the opportunity to become NPs because their CNS positions were declared redundant due to perceived lack of cost-effectiveness, only to find this role being replaced with case managers, clinical resource nurses, and others. Registered nurses working at the bedside have repeatedly been replaced by registered practical nurses and patient service workers. Current professional and public discourse is replete with controversy regarding the need for NPs, who are being encouraged to promote themselves as a cheaper alternative to other health care providers (American Academy of Nurse Practitioners, 2010; CNA, 2002). The use of physician assistants as alternatives to NPs is another current discourse that has emerged on the Canadian scene; it is an appealing option for physicians, who retain control over their activities, and for institutions, as PAs are paid less. Therefore, is there a possibility that the fear of replacement connects with the discourse on owing something more to the organization? Owing not only implies that one has an obligation or duty to give back something of equal value in return for something received; inherently, the sense of obligation creates a sense of being owned or of belonging to another in an instrumental and economic way.

Why does the organization believe that NPs owe the system more than what they already do in the clinical domain of their practice? Does this reflect the overall devaluing of hands-on care that arises from the nursing role? Current NP discourses have resulted in the NP being constituted as an object of nature and therefore understood metaphorically as a tool or instrument within the health care system to be used efficiently and effectively. Charles Taylor (1991b, p. 5), in The Malaise of Modernity, argued that when a society is redesigned on the values and beliefs of individualism and autonomy, instrumental reason becomes the yardstick by which success is measured. Consequently, individuals become vulnerable "to being treated as raw materials or instruments for our projects." Heidegger (1977, pp. 14–23) argued that technology imposes a particular sorting, ordering, commanding, and disposing of nature and humans. It seeks to unlock, transform, store up, and distribute concealed energy from nature and humans and order it into a "standing reserve." The result of this stockpiling is that modern technology orders everything and everyone to stand by, to be always ready to be used and to be on call for further doing.

Heidegger (1977) further argued that the essence of modern technology is to seek to order everything so as to achieve more and more flexibility and efficiency: "Expediting is always itself directed toward furthering something else, i.e. toward driving on to the maximum yield at the minimum expense" (p.15). Heidegger concluded that whatever "stands by in the sense of standing-reserve no longer stands over against us as object" (p. 17). Viewed from this perspective, NPs, for example, are not individuals who engage in meeting patients' needs as worked through in the NP–patient relationship but are manipulated by the system to do its work. In essence, NPs become a resource to be not only used but also enhanced. "Man, who no longer conceals his character of being the most important raw material, is also drawn into this process" (Heidegger, quoted in Dreyfus, 1993, p. 306).

In contemporary times, NPs have come to be regarded as machines or tools to be scrutinized in terms of possible uses and efficiencies within the workplace. This discourse allows NPs to be thought of in terms of what their role is, but not in a way that provides a space for knowing who NPs are, what their interior life is, and what it means to be an NP. In becoming an object, the NP as a tool has been separated from the whole person. The full measure of what NPs have to offer their patients has failed to arise in the discourse and therefore remains invisible. This way of being may be interpreted as less valuable, and only activities that are identified in dialogue with others are perceived as having enough value to be retained in the system. The dominant discourse, for instance, has not made visible the time and skill that it takes to be physically, personally, and existentially available to the patient. In many cases, the NPs' "hidden riches" (Dreyfus, 1992, p. 177) have failed to surface even at the institutional level.

There are "technological traps" (Bergum, 2003, p. 123) inherent in viewing and being viewed from an instrumental and economic viewpoint. One trap is the power of technology to direct human action. Danger arises when individuals become mere objects, managed and controlled as the means to accomplish technological ends (Gadow, 1994), because they begin to view themselves from this perspective. No wonder some NPs feel like puppets whose movements are controlled by the whims and fancy of others. The puppeteers, or external force, such as nursing management and physicians, can force an adaptation and flexibility that results in an experience of being more controlled rather than being more in control.

The puppet analogy carries a significance that is deeper than may first appear and can be closely associated with the power of technology. The word *puppet* is derived from the Latin word *pupa*, meaning "girl" (Barnhart, 1988) or "doll." Since the sixteenth century, *puppet* has been defined as a particular kind of doll that acts on a stage under human direction. Similarly, the word *pupil*, derived from the Latin word *pūpilla*, meaning "minor," was understood to be a person who could see herself reflected in miniature, like a doll, in the eye of the other. The Anglo-Norman word *pupille*, meaning an orphan child in the care of a guardian, also descended from this Latin word.

Through history, both women and orphans have often been perceived as chattel, property of others to be used as cheap and expendable labour, objects in service for instrumental and economic ends. Does this also apply to nursing, a predominantly female profession with a strong history of being dominated by others? If it does, some NPs may see themselves in others' eyes as smaller, minor, and consequently of less significance, than those who gaze upon them. From this instrumental and economic viewpoint, it is unsurprising to discover that although many NPs acknowledge being good nurse practitioners, in being pulled to be more they often question themselves: *Am I good enough? Am I doing a good enough job? If I'm not perceived as doing enough of the work, and I'm not doing the CNS or advanced nursing practice role, again am I not good* enough? So, as secure as NPs can sound in the clinical component of their role, they have many insecurities.

A second trap is the effect of technical language (Bergum and Dosseter, 2003). Labels such as "physician extenders" and "physician replacements" carry not only a sense of objectness but also a negative social connotation. Bergum and Dosseter found that moral language is lost when we engage in this form of discourse. These labels evoke no sense of nurse, the practice of nursing, or the commitment that NPs embody as a result of belonging to the nursing world. One NP made the following observation about being called a mini-physician and physician replacement:

> I think it negates the whole nursing side of it, the whole nursing background piece that we all bring into the nurse practitioner role, and that encompasses all the human compassion aspect that we talked about. It all gets negated. Because when you use the descriptor "physician," you're automatically thinking more medical model than, "Oh, you take care of families as well as the patients."

The third trap is the effect of the polarization of self that this view tends to foster (Bergum and Dossester, 2003). For example, when nursing administrators engage in discourse that dichotomizes the domains of the NP role into direct clinical care (physician-replacement activities) and education, leadership, and research (nursing activities), NPs are once again encouraged to experience themselves as being a polarization of opposites.

But who "owns" the NPs? Certainly, NPs who have found the perfect fit observe that those who hold the purse strings have the power to determine the expectations for the role. For some, the salary is controlled entirely by nursing, while for others, medicine and nursing hold equal shares. For example, one NP shared that as a result of the clinical workload associated with managing the inpatient population, clinics, and all phone calls for the service, she had negotiated with her nursing manager to "give up" one of the subspecialty clinics within the service. However she stated that, "The physicians said that since they pay part of my salary that I needed to go back there. I didn't really have choice."

As importantly, many NPs have also mentioned that they are indebted to the physicians with whom they work. Physicians determine both the nature of the safety line, with its inherent promise to keep both the patient and the NP from harm, and the nature of the clinical work in which NPs are allowed to engage. The degree of autonomy and the scope of clinical practice are contingent on the physicians with whom they work, for they approve the medical directives (or their equivalent) in the institution and then delegate the types of patients for whom NPs may care. This is the paradoxical nature of power. While NPs attain the power to belong, to be a certain person, to claim a place with the legitimacy of membership (if only on the margins), they also experience the vulnerability of belonging to, identifying with, and being members of some communities that contribute to defining who they are and thus have a hold on them (Wenger, 1998). The tension between the identification and negotiability inherent in power as well as its richness and complexity is thus revealed.

In contrast, some NPs experience the tension of being pulled to be more as a welcome opportunity that needs to be seized, despite warnings from other NPs that it will deflect them from the role's essential work. For example, one NP recalled that it was her medical mentor who raised the idea that she consider her role in developing nurses professionally. She was both surprised that a physician would use those words and embarrassed that it took a physician to encourage her to become involved in what she envisioned to be part of her role. However, she interpreted his remark to mean that she was now competent in the clinical management of her patients and therefore was ready to take on other challenges. Knowing that she could not engage in additional responsibilities without protected time, she seized this opportunity to negotiate with both the medical staff and the nursing manager for one day per week away from direct patient-care responsibilities. As she noted, although she felt blessed to work with such a supportive group, it was her responsibility to make it happen.

Some NPs become restless with the purely clinical nature of their role, a feeling that emerges at the time that their clinical acumen has become more honed. The paradox of their jobs is that the narrowness and tight focus of their specialty, although overwhelming during the early part of their career, eventually becomes a source of frustration. While the routine nature of their clinical work brings into being a sense of comfort and confidence, it also creates the need and desire for new challenges; they begin to re-experience the call to stretch themselves in new and different ways. Feeling bored, under-stimulated, or in a rut, some NPs hanker after new and different opportunities that will help them to be more challenged or to use some of their advanced skills, such as project work and research. Some are being pulled to be more because they believe that only in the enactment of other advanced nursing practice competencies will they be viewed as more than physician replacements, because the possibility of being more connected with nurses lies in making more of a difference to the nursing profession. For these NPs, the search for the perfect fit has still not been achieved.

Some NPs have a clear sense of direction about how they should proceed with their journey, and so being pulled to be more is not experienced as a turbulent period. Others, however, may struggle to identify where to explore next. All they can acknowledge is that the pull to be more exists.

I'd like to have some very specific interest or interests that I can work on besides the clinical, and whether it's to be able to teach that portion of it or do research on it, I'm not sure. But I'm feeling a need to try and find a focus, something that really interests me. And I do like some of the discharge stuff, and maybe I will pursue some of that discharge planning, but I really want something a little bit more concrete too, something maybe not quite physiological, but along those lines. So right now it's mostly clinical, but I'm hoping that it'll be a more well-rounded role at some point. But I'm floundering; I don't know.

Some NPs feel an internal pull to be more, experienced as the need to expand more, to become more complete. They are ready to tackle more either clinically or in the other components of the advanced practice role. They want to develop and use new knowledge and skills, or embed the knowledge and skills that they possess from previous roles into their NP practice. If they encounter resistance to taking on these challenges, the pull to be more may cause tension that for some becomes a source of frustration to be circumnavigated.

The major barrier obstructing NPs' attempts to move beyond the clinical component of their role is lack of administrative and medical support, a finding consistent with studies that have explored factors that hinder NP role performance (Kilpatrick et al., 2010; Reay, Golden-Biddle, and GermAnn, 2003; van Soeren and Micevski, 2001). Resistance from physicians presents itself in the form of refusal to grant time away from patient-care activities. Nursing management is perceived as silent on the issue, ineffective in lobbying on their behalf, or lacking in an appreciation of the potential for NP role development. One NP found herself constantly stalled by the "can't do" philosophy of leadership within her organization. Physician priorities and lack of flexibility with how clinical practice could work take precedence over the vision of how NPs can contribute differently to the organization. These NPs struggle with their inability to negotiate their role description or enactment of the role as they desire it to be: "Clinical takes precedence, so whenever you're at work you're at the beck and call of the unit. They can call me or page me anytime if there's a shortage of hands and that's where I'm expected to be. Everything else takes second place to clinical. And I just would like someday for it to be more than clinical."

The yearning for more is heightened when NPs glimpse what this could mean for themselves and others. One described an opportunity she had had to provide a series of in-services to recovery-room nurses who had found that they lacked the knowledge needed to be confident about and comfortable with implementing a new pharmacological treatment. Despite having to fit the teaching sessions into the middle of a busy day, she really enjoyed knowing that the nurses now had a better appreciation of the medical condition as a whole and could safely manage the patients' episodes. She acknowledged that the patients, nurses, and she would benefit highly if she could only be involved in more teaching, but she was unsure if she could get beyond the barriers imposed by the clinical challenges.

Unable to do what was originally envisioned for the role, another NP described her ongoing, albeit occasional, struggle with being an NP as "sometimes feeling like a go-fer" for the physicians, all the while hearing the managers say that the NPs should be doing research and they should be setting aside time to publish. Unable to accomplish either of these in her role, she admitted that sometimes she felt that she had not met the expectations of the role and wished she could do a better job. Under these circumstances, some NPs engage in other domains of practice on their own time, often working seventy- to eighty-hour workweeks, while others search for different employment opportunities or simply live with the tension. One NP found that the best way to compromise and fit in some of these other activities is by presenting at a yearly conference outside the hospital setting:

The role is called NP/CNS. So, of course, what I've described is mostly nurse practitioner stuff, and by rights, that's only supposed to take 80 percent of my time. *We're supposed to have 20 percent, or equivalent to one day a week, doing the CNS part. Unfortunately there isn't time for that. Management recognizes that they would like us to do more in the CNS part. They're the ones who pay our salary and they're not getting the added nursing value, as I've heard some upper-management people say. But, by the same token, the surgeons have become quite accustomed to looking on us as being their assistants, so it's hard to explain to them why you're not going to attend to that patient issue because you want to work on something else. So the something else doesn't happen, at least with my role. I just have to sneak it in in other ways. . . . It would be nice to be able to wear both hats, but unless I can negotiate one non-clinical day a week, it just won't happen. I'm already working ten-hour days. I just can't fit the time in. So I miss out on it.*

Lack of support can also come in the form of missing mentorship opportunities for advanced practice nursing competencies for which many NPs have limited to no knowledge and skill. As a result, these NPs re-experience feelings of incompetence, non-confidence, and discomfort with being an educator, researcher, leader, or change agent. They acknowledge that they flounder and shy away from some or all of these activities:

I think it's because our programs, although they have research in them, they don't really; and even subsequent to getting the job and going through your orientation, it isn't on how to do research. It's on how to take care of the patients, and that was where your skill set was developed. . . . Even though I have the theory, it's a whole different ball of wax to implement it, and I believe that one of the reasons that we don't do research is that we don't know that much about research, we're not really skilled in it. . . . If we had somebody who had met with us regularly and helped us develop our ideas, not just say, "Well go off with your idea and come back to me," because . . . you don't feel skilled in that area, and so you just keep feeling really tentative, and you can't really get going. . . . It's not that I'm really averse to research but I feel like I don't really know what I'm doing.

In fact, under these circumstances, some NPs revisit a number of the feelings associated with being adrift. Uncertain what they want to do, where they want to go, or how to get there, they say that not being quite the beginners anymore but not yet the experts is a frustrating place to be. As one NP observed, when one is a beginner, permission is granted to ask questions and be offered advice. When one is an expert, neither seems to be necessary. Having proven themselves in the clinical arena but not in the other advanced practice competencies, NPs may find themselves without anyone to foster their ongoing growth and development:

They are NP experts because they don't have to put so much time and energy into the clinical every day; it doesn't take as much out of them and they have the time and energy to do other things. . . . But I find that . . . some of the middle-grounders like me aren't in a position to do that right now. . . . We need the office time or protected time off the unit to be able to pursue other things, other interests besides LPs and whatever, because, although we're able to do the clinical, it still may take us some more time than the experts, plus we don't yet know how to do the other parts of the job. That takes a lot of time too. . . . And I think the director tends to lump us together probably more than she should . . . and then if you point that out to her, "Oh yes, you're right," and then it is beginners and experts. Well, there are not just beginners and experts; there's the whole in-between.

Even when the pull to be more is internally motivated, NPs observe that it may be strongly opposed by the pull to stay entirely immersed in direct clinical practice. The allure that advanced clinical management of the patient may have for them, particularly when most of them have been searching to be more in control, more visible, more challenged, and more connected with patients and families while performing hands-on care, is not difficult to understand. One NP articulated that the type of focus that results from prescribing, ordering diagnostic tests, and engaging in a more detailed level of physical assessment "is sexier, more powerful." As she admitted there is authoritarian and implied hierarchical power in the term *physician order*, and although she recognized that *power over* is detrimental to nursing, she also readily acknowledged that when a nurse has that power, it is "very easy to get sucked into it." This back-and-forth pull is a struggle. She noted that the power associated with these entitlements of the role may lead NPs away from that which has been intended or envisioned for the role: "Being in a position of the one that people go to puts the NP in a position of power and you can choose to use that to keep yourself up there or you can choose to share it. But it is somewhat of a personal choice." This NP's admission of temptation with power's "dark side" reveals the psychological burden NPs may bear that is associated with the power to act in the clinical sphere as garnered in being an NP. But the desire that some NPs have to make more of a difference by bearing and sharing power, rather than wielding it, is also revealed: some NPs use their power as a matter of conscious choice to escape its constitutive danger.

Living with *either/or* is promoted when nursing management and others engage in discourse that presents patient-care activities as medical functions belonging solely to the NP role, while the other advanced practice competencies represent the nursing orientation to the role. NPs attempt to reconcile the ideals of their education and expectations that emerge from the discourse of others with the realities of the context of their practice and their personal desires for the perfect fit. How do NPs experience their professional selves as they live with or journey through the tension experienced in being pulled to be more?

Being a Wearer of Two Hats

This time in the NPs' journey is, once again, experienced as a time of living with a polarization of opposites — or, what NPs referred to as the wearing of two hats, the "NP hat" of direct patient care and the "CNS hat" of leadership, research, and education.

Right now I mostly have my medical or NP hat on, but I guess I'd like to be able to do some research and be a principal investigator . . . and I think there's room for expansion in leadership as far as being involved in more decision-making as far as nursing within the hospital. . . . I'd like to be able to wear the CNS hat too.

Actually, the CNS/NP title is an interesting one. . . . When I have the NP hat on, it's basically very physically and psychosocially oriented. . . . I find the CNS hat allows me to have a little bit of time for research, which is something that I wish I could do more of.

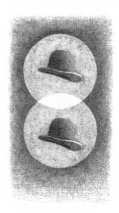

FIG. 3. *Hats 1.* Courtesy Tom Phillips and The Folio Society.

Time is experienced as being diverted from one role to another; the direct-practice activities are sacrificed to the other advanced-practice competencies or vice versa. For some, this polarization results from a resistance to engage in all competencies of advanced practice when the search for more has ended and the perfect fit has been found. For others, the polarization results from a lack of knowledge or skill in how to perform in these components of the role, while the call to find the perfect fit, to experience more, remains only partially fulfilled. This dichotomy is further enhanced by job titles such as NP, NP/CNS, and CNS/NP. These titles are not designated provincially, regionally, or institutionally. In fact, it is not uncommon to find all three titles within a single institution. Some NPs carry all of them at different points in their careers, as a result of either a move to another institution or a change in expectation for their role within a single institution.

> NP/CNS is the title here and it's a bit of a misnomer because we're certainly more NP than we are CNS although we keep trying. . . . And I'm not sure who came up with the title NP/CNS. The title has gone through many evolutions in this organization. It used to be CNS/NP and then some time over the last four or five years it switched around. When you look at our job description . . . certain proportions are supposed to be devoted to clinical, education, research, and professional development of the nursing staff.

Titles have the capacity to either constrain or expand what NPs do by identifying expectations with regard to the boundaries of their scope of practice and sphere of influence. For example, the singular NP title has the tendency to limit the vision for the NP position, since the dominant discourse associated with this title recognizes or acknowledges only one aspect of the role and speaks to it in terms of medicine. The title eliminates and devalues the other aspects of advanced nursing practice, which are either lost or buried within the title, thus making these aspects of the role invisible. It seems that an appreciation for the contributions that NPs can make under the umbrella of "advanced nursing practice" has yet to be translated into the singular NP title at the level where NPs live their work. If barriers, such as time constraints and lack of resources, also exist which inhibit the expansion of those boundaries, NPs are forced to enact the discourse, which serves only to reinforce the other's hegemonic view of their role. Consequently, in a catch-22, the title defines the space in which NPs live and practice. On the other hand, the titles NP/CNS and CNS/NP suggest that there are two different sets of role functions brought together to be carried out by one individual. The specific placement of the two roles within the title often signifies the dominant commitment of NPs' time and perhaps what is most valued by the organization or the NP. The title is subsequently viewed as a dual job, with the proportion of time allocated to each adding up to a full-time job.

If we are to look at the role itself, because they put the NP first, that's the big clinical chunk. The academic and the research and the professional development come as part of the clinical nurse specialist role, and so that takes a much lesser role. So probably 75 to 80 percent of our time is clinical and only 20 to 25 percent is the CNS hat we put on. Others have a 50–50 split, but it doesn't work well when you're by yourself and you have to do all the clinical work. So really I wear the NP hat most of the time.

Ironically, while some NPs lobby to have their title changed from NP to NP/CNS in order to legitimize or justify the time they spend, or want to spend, involved in the other components of advanced nursing practice, other NPs argue that the singular NP title accurately reflects the focus of the role. Although these NPs are being pulled to be more by nursing management, the singular NP title legitimizes their belief that research, education, and leadership activities belong to the CNS role. If they have found the perfect fit, the singular title allows them to justify living within the perceived boundaries that this title appears to imply.

Each title, with its succinctness, portability, potential persistence, and focusing effects, gives NPs certain experiences and informs their communities of practice about what they should pay attention to. In other words, the title becomes a form of reification. But the evocative power of these titles is also double-edged, because they do not capture the richness of the NPs' lived experiences. Rather, the titles have, in some cases, appropriated what NPs do in very misleading ways. The titles have gained concreteness, which becomes something that both the NPs and others refer to, strive for, appeal to, and use or misuse in arguments. In fact, the focus on the title may become a substitute for what was never intended to be reflected in the first place. Becoming an NP, CNS/NP, or NP/CNS is both taking on the label and giving the label specific meanings through participation in practice.

Because they are pioneers, NPs have experienced fluidity in their role, which may have impeded coordination, created apprehension about potential misalignments, or resulted in confusion and misunderstandings. Yet this same fluidity has allowed for interactive negotiation, as well as improvisation and creativity, which is the very nature of advanced practice nursing roles: dynamic and continually evolving in response to the changing contexts and health care needs of patients, organizations, and health care systems (CNA, 2008). This fluidity permits NPs within their communities of practice to seize moments and see opportunities that would not have otherwise been revealed. Thus titles as a form of reification may reinforce or anchor the specificities or expectations of the NPs' practice, but too much reliance may be placed on the anchoring, at the expense of the emergence of all the possibilities for being and becoming an NP.

The paradox of the current titling discourse is that it separates the CNS and NP roles, resulting in NPs seeing the various advanced practice competencies as diametrically opposed. Although they may participate in some or all of the competencies at this time in their journey, they perceive themselves as performing two jobs. At the same time, the split title legitimizes NPs' engagement in all of the role competencies when there is external resistance to their doing so, thus opening the possibility for some to experience a transformational journey to unification of competencies. The allotment of proportions of time, even if only on paper, may also serve to marginalize aspects of the NPs' work or their desire for more.

NPs' stories reveal the relationship between the enactment of the role and their identity as NPs. Some, particularly if they have found a fit in being an NP, identify more with the dominant focus of the role, which is associated with direct patient care. They refer to themselves as NPs and are disconnected from the other competencies: "I think we are nurse practitioners and we may dabble in or do some of the clinical nurse specialist traditional role, but we're predominantly a nurse practitioner." Although they may participate in other activities, such as education, committee work, or research, these activities are experienced as pieces of the job to be added on to their NP responsibilities.

The titling creates an expectation of who we think we are based on the tasks, rather than how it is and the philosophy with which we come to the job. And I think some of that comes from the way we are viewed by other nurses. It's quite often been viewed or seen that we're physician assistants and we're not fulfilling a nursing role, and that's come from administration in the building. And I don't think they have a good understanding of what we do or how we do it, and maybe we haven't presented that well to them either. But they think that in being an NP we're doing more the physician role

than the nurse role. . . . Even though we probably have more nurse
practitioners in this building than any other hospital in the country,
there is still misunderstanding by administration and nursing
administration about what we do and who we are.

Staying clinically focused and clinically driven is identified as the heart of being a nurse practitioner; otherwise NPs "are not different from the clinical nurse specialist." Yet tension exists when NPs are unable to add or combine the other role competencies to ensure that they will be set apart from "the physician assistant medical model." As a result of these various discourses and the tension perceived, NPs may even experience the dichotomy of identities as being split and straddling two worlds. "Gretchen," who held the title NP/CNS, described her role as spending 60 to 70 percent of [her] time as an acute-care nurse practitioner and the other 30 to 40 percent of her time as really wearing the CNS hat, a time allotment she deemed fair. She related multiple examples of her participation in informal and formal educational initiatives with nursing staff and students, the development and implementation of support programs focused on the spiritual and sexual needs of her patients within her subspecialty of practice, and the initiation of and participation in research projects prompted by questions arising from her clinical practice. Yet she acknowledged that she still feels schizophrenic.

Gretchen recognized that the advantage of having the NP hat attached to her name allows her to create opportunities not heretofore afforded. For example, she was able to initiate a joint paediatric-adult clinic for paediatric patients transitioning to the adult sector within her subspecialty, and the identification of research questions that "really came out of wearing [her] NP hat." She acknowledged that she would not want to give up the ability to manage the patients' symptoms in a timely manner or the procedures through which she can attend to the patients' and

families' issues and worries in a way that is different from the
physicians. However, Gretchen worked with a team in which she
perceived that members saw her only as an assistant to the physician, assisting with physical exams and performing procedures.
As a result, she felt like an NP as opposed to a CNS, although she
also acknowledged that being an NP had been a good fit for more
than five years. In the following, Gretchen reveals the ongoing
dialectic in which she is engaged and the unresolved turmoil:

But am I wearing my CNS hat or am I wearing my NP hat now?
What is it that I'm doing in all of this? Part of me feels it's more
the CNS role. So if I get going with the [new] program, work with
them one-on-one, is that the CNS role or the NP role? I'm just
struggling with that right now actually at this point in my career.
But in some ways I am always doing the medical piece too. . . .
And where do I want to go? What do I need to do to feel comfortable
going to work every day? . . . Maybe I'll be able to really integrate
the nursing piece, the CNS piece, with this other piece. I've struggled,
no, really gone out of my way, to really maintain and develop some
skills in terms of research and some other aspects of the CNS role.
So I've really tried to wear two hats basically at the same time.
But I think I've gotten to the point where I'm not sure that I want
to continue in the acute-care nurse practitioner piece of it. Or, if I
do want to continue, how should it look? . . . So I don't know if it's
just me or if other people struggle with this too. Do I need to look
at the role a little bit differently and see how I can be happier in
that role?

Gretchen believes that when she finally chooses between the NP
hat and the CNS hat, the tension with which she has been living
will be released. However, there is a fallacy in this assumption.
The tension experienced by all NPs in being pulled to be more
is a central tension about the expression of numerous obligations

involving confrontations of disparate viewpoints. These differing expectations for practice give rise to clashes of intentions, in which NPs, nursing management, physicians, staff nurses, and others assign motivational aims to the other(s) from their own respective understandings. Gretchen is striving to reconcile disparities she cannot escape. Both individual and collective work must be done during this transitional and transformational journey.

Do NPs have to choose one or the other hat? Must they live with the tension forever if they choose not to give up either? Perhaps not. A title, and the understanding of what the title means, even a negotiated meaning, is transacted within the politics of relationships. NPs working within their various communities of practice are not self-contained entities. In any community, people grow and develop within larger contexts — historical, social, cultural, and institutional — with specific resources and constraints. However, geographical proximity to other NPs, the network through which information flows, the presence of a job description, and even belonging to a particular organization is not sufficient to relieve the tension of living with a polarity of opposites. Further, the NPs' individual responses to their conditions hinder or facilitate the transition through the time of being pulled to be more. Just as NPs gradually experience an inner transformation as they journey from being adrift to being an NP, some NPs embrace the tension created by the two constitutive practices of the "CNS hat" and the "NP hat," and learn the delicate balance of combining both to work toward the larger quest of being more.

This is not to say that communities of practice are exempt from creating supportive and nurturing environments that are sensitive to this transitional and transformative process. However, NPs need to continue the journey in order to find a way to reconcile the tension experienced at this time. Some NPs use this tension as an opportunity to continue their journey in search of the perfect fit.

If I had my choice I would love to be able to able to have time to develop in-services and then do a couple of teaching sessions on the floor to help keep the nurses current with what's going on with their patients. Then I could satisfy needs of other staff members as well, and hopefully indirectly then provide better patient care. And although I mentioned before that research intimidates me because I've never done it, I would certainly like to work with somebody on their projects and maybe that would open some windows for me. They would be opportunities that I would like to see happen. So I dream, and if you don't have a dream you're not going to get anywhere. . . . You know, you learn so many things that you tend to go in one way or the other before you really decide what you want to do and who you are. And so I don't think I'm at the end of the road in terms of expanding my role. There's so much more to who I am as an NP that has yet to be explored.

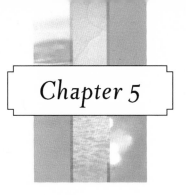

Chapter 5

Being More

With new opportunities for learning and an ongoing dialectic engagement, NPs may continue their journey, through being pulled to be more to live the experience of being more. In being more, NPs undergo another inner transformation, in which they gradually unify the various advanced nursing practice role competencies such that increasing the level of participation in any one competency does not dispense with any of the others; on the contrary, the requirement to participate in the other competencies is increased. Why do some NPs experience this transformation while others do not?

Wenger (1998, p. 176) told the story of two stonecutters who are asked what they are doing. One responds, "I am cutting this stone in a perfectly square shape." The other responds, "I am building a cathedral." As Wenger pointed out, "Both answers are correct and meaningful, but they reflect different relations to the world." The difference does not imply that one person is a better stonecutter than the other, as far as holding the chisel is concerned. At the level of enactment, both may be doing exactly the same thing, but each stonecutter's experience of what he is doing and his sense of self in doing it is different. This difference is a function of imagination.

If NPs' journeys are viewed from the perspective of this analogy, they differ as a function of the imagined vision of the perfect fit for which each initiated his or her respective journey. Given that each journey and way of being is different — not better or worse — each NP may learn and understand very different things from the same activities, and journey to very different places, both personally and professionally.

Wenger (1998, p. 176) viewed imagination as "a process of expanding our self by transcending our time and space and creating new images of the world and ourselves." In this sense, imagination is looking at the NP role and seeing the possibility of the perfect fit. It is an NP envisioning quality of care for her patients as "one-stop care for individuals . . . that includes health promotion as well as tertiary-level care . . . and being provided outside the walls of a large tertiary-care centre because not all clients necessarily like coming to hospitals for their care." It is an NP hearing about a health care issue in his or her own setting, knowing that issue is experienced by thousands of patients or nurses around the world, and then partnering with other professionals from around the world to find creative solutions through the sharing of expertise. It is an NP envisioning the use of her artistic talents to research and establish an art therapy program to help ease her patients' suffering. It is NPs seeing themselves as "being able to work with patients and staff in the same moment."

Wenger (1998, p. 177) said that imagination, used in this context, "emphasizes the creative process of producing new images and of generating new relations through time and space that become constitutive of the self." It involves a different kind of work of the self — one that concerns the production of images of the self and of the world that transcend or reach beyond direct engagement. Rather than being a purely individual process, it is anchored in social interactions and communal experiences. "It is a mode of belonging that always involves the social world to expand the scope of reality and identity" (Wenger, 1998, p. 178). "Being able to be creative with a group of people," noted one NP, "goes a long way in terms of feeling happy in my job and growth and satisfaction." One NP used an example to explore the meaning of being creative in her role, what she described as problem-solving with others and identifying issues that are significant for patients and families that others have yet to recognize or explore. Unable to help families who turned to her for advice on how to best manage their loved ones' fatigue during cancer treatment, and because there was little research on this health care issue, she presented to members of her interprofessional team the idea of engaging in research to address this problem. Over the course of several months, the group generated potential research questions and ideas for moving the project forward. The NP then used the national oncology organization to search for an opportunity to work with experienced nursing researchers: "I became a co-investigator on the project — and that's fine because that's how you learn — and I obtained a scholarship from the Oncology Nursing Society, a novice researcher mentor award. . . . So we've done two studies in relation to fatigue with this population. It's gotten to the point where we've developed a brochure on healthy lifestyles in patients with cancer and I've included a section in there on how you manage fatigue."

Imagination as anchored in social processes is evident when NPs identify the Athenas in their personal and professional lives, individuals who are the wings beneath their feet, or when they describe the joy, satisfaction, and sense of being empowered and enriched when working in open and receptive "can-do" and "why not?" environments. Then again, imagination is stifled, disconnected, and ineffective when NPs work with naysayers and obstructionists or practice within "top-down" or "follow the rules" environments.

Imagining one's practice as a continuing history is difficult if one lives with the fear of replacement. Conceiving new developments, exploring alternatives, or envisioning possible futures is problematic if one does not have a sense of belonging to one's local community of practice or to the broader social system in which one operates. If NPs do not perceive that they have power over their own energies or the capacity to inspire self or others, their imaginations may become narrowed and diminished. However, the imagining of who one is, what one can become, and what one can do helps to prevent the NP from being only that which has been imagined by others.

In being more, NPs discover how they grow again in their understanding of what nursing practice is and what their practice can be. They even begin to have a fresh view of others in their roles, and this recognition brings about a new valuing. This is illustrated in a well-known quote from Marcel Proust (1999, p. 803): "The real voyage of discovery consists not in seeking new landscapes, but in seeing with new eyes."

Part of the growth process and maturation of being in this new role was, by working with others in a new way, I learned about valuing. So, for example, I learned more about the respiratory therapists — who they are, what they come to the table with, and what attributes they bring to the situation that we're working together in. It's sort of that whole re-education about the value of other professions. . . . And so that first experience of working outside that [nursing] box . . . [I saw] that there are different ways of doing things, and that one way is not always the right way, and no one person has control, and you can't have control over everyone else either. It was just to see how much value we all have and that we all bring what we're experts at to the game, and then we have a much better game.

In this time and place of being more, NPs continually experience new ways of "building on their nursing practice," "always trying to get to a point to be ready to test new waters," and "setting new directions and new horizons." Being more is about imagining how to use all their accumulated knowledge and experiences gained through a lifetime of nursing to constantly further this nursing role. It is about imagining a role that is not just clinical but also an advanced practice role that sees "clinical nursing in a bigger, broader sense" and provides the "opportunity to integrate so many different aspects into one practice," many of which have been developed during previous career paths.

But [being an NP] is also about being able to bring all of the experiences that I've had throughout my career, being able to work with a variety of people, being able to make a difference at the bedside, and also being able to do some of those other advanced practice roles — being able to go to conferences, present, publish, do research, mentor colleagues, being able to interact with different people, different organizations. I think all of those things are really critical, for me, to the NP role. Because you have to not just make a difference at the bedside, but you have to make a difference to the staff that you work with. I think you need to influence the physicians that you work with, and you need to influence the broader nursing community. Maybe you can't do it all the time with other demands, but at some point you need to be able to say, Okay, I need to put energy into and contribute to moving nursing practice forward. And it's neat because the NP role allows me to do everything, has the potential to do everything, if you want to go on that road.

In being more, NPs reconcile the dichotomy of being NPs and CNSs. They "blend the CNS component with the NP component . . . to make a true advanced practice role." Undeniably, they struggle to juggle or balance their time, but time and workload create the tension, not the sense of being split. These NPs have one identity made up of many components, in a mixture that is unique to each of them, just as others' identities are unique to them as individuals.

Perhaps the NP who has made this reconciliation is most similar to Janus, the Roman god of gates, doors, doorways, beginnings, and endings. Janus is most commonly depicted with two faces looking in opposite directions and has frequently been used to symbolize transitions such as the progression from past to future, one condition to another, one vision to another, one world to another, and adolescence and adulthood (Hamilton, 1940). Hence, this figure has been representative of the middle ground, or in-between time and place, reminiscent of Aoki's (2005, p. 318) image of "crossing" between East and West, a "generative space of possibilities, a space wherein . . . newness emerges." It may be that these NPs find themselves as part of "a story of unfinalized hybridity, of unceasing attempts to bring together disparate parts, respecting their otherness . . . but believing in a harmony among these parts" (Frank, 2004, p. 105). Perhaps, as Stuart Hall (1990, p. 223) stated, "there is the recognition of a necessary hetero-geneity and diversity . . . a conception of 'identity' which lives with and through, not despite difference." Perhaps NPs' renewed identities, as Hall describes identity, "are those which are con-stantly producing and reproducing themselves anew, through transformation and difference." (p. 223)

Being an Advanced Practitioner

Below are three NPs' stories. These stories bring forth each NP's unique practice and the work in which she is engaged, based on her imagination of what it means to be an advanced practitioner and thus who she is as an NP. What is illuminated through these three stories, both explicitly and implicitly, is that being more in being advanced practitioners gives meaning to these NPs' practices and renews their sense of identity; they have discovered the perfect fit during the transformation to being more as experienced through being an advanced practitioner. All advanced nursing practice competencies are viewed as inseparable and mutually constitutive, and their complementarity gives the NP role its richness, dynamism, and uniqueness, all of which are also beautifully illustrated in the three representations of two hats by the illustrator Tom Phillips. Ultimately, NPs identify themselves as encompassing all of these competencies and are seen this way by others in their communities of practice.

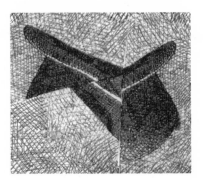

FIG. 4. *Hats 2.* Courtesy Tom Phillips and The Folio Society.

The first story concerns "Jenny," an NP working in a critical-care environment. Her designated title is NP and, despite numerous battles such as unemployment, workload demands — "in reality, the clinical component is 99 percent of my job, but part of the difficulty is that nobody knows that there's another 25 percent of my job, even though I keep telling them over and over again" — bedside nursing resistance, and lack of administrative support, she believes that she has finally found the perfect fit in being more. For her, an NP is part of the big umbrella of advanced practice nursing in which CNSs and NPs must work together, albeit with a different division of workload. Jenny and the program's CNS identify day-to-day issues that frustrate them or which they see as problems that have global impact on the program. Having completed several research projects and having published and presented at national or international conferences at least once each year, Jenny has established that research, in partnership with the CNS, is now an integral part of her role.

For example, Jenny and her colleague perceived that there were unnecessary delays in endotracheal tube (ETT) extubations, which resulted in an increased incidence of ventilator-associated pneumonias, prolonged lengths of stay in the intensive care unit, and increased costs to the health care system. Jenny noted that, "an NP doesn't have a zillion hours to develop proposals and go to Ethics, and so we worked together." Both were involved in the literature review and research proposal development, but the CNS wrote the formal proposal and research ethics application. Jenny approached nurses in the clinical area to "to help out with data collection, to try to bring them into thinking about nursing research, maybe get them excited about it and want to be part of improving practice." Both provided education to the unit staff on the benefits of early extubation based on scientific and local evidence.

Jenny and her partner subsequently undertook a post-extubation evaluation and found that they had made a significant improvement in timely ETT extubations. Early extubation also reduced the use of sedatives by half, thus saving the system $15,000 annually. As a result of the success of this clinically-driven research project,

Jenny and the CNS became involved in improving the unit's pain assessment and documentation, and developed research proposals related to oral care and diabetic management, the latter project being an outcome of Jenny's participation on a hospital quality assurance committee for the practices of insulin and diabetic management. As a result of embedding nursing research, education, and quality management activities into her practice, Jenny observed:

> The nurses see me as a role model, and maybe I've even been a mentor to a few nurses — because we have had probably about 10 nurses in our ICU actually go back into the master's program because they actually want to do this role. And they see me as somebody who has some knowledge who they can approach to ask questions or who they see as being able to facilitate their learning as well. I love to do one-on-one teaching at the bedside with them, and a lot of times it happens when things are happening with their patients and they're getting orders for this and that and sometimes when they are new or less experienced, they don't always feel comfortable asking physicians because they're scared or it's a power thing, but they feel comfortable saying to me, "Well why exactly are we doing this, what is the reason and what is the outcome hopefully going to be?" So it makes you feel good about yourself as a nurse and as a person to be able to do all these things, as well as have hands on all the time.

The second story is told by "Colleen," an NP who became tired of being told by senior nursing administration that she "could not have or do everything" in nursing. She was pushed to make up her mind about whether she wanted to be a clinician, a researcher, an educator, or a manager. Having wrestled with the question *What do you want to do?* she finally decided that she was "just going to have it all." For Colleen, being an advanced practitioner means doing everything, all the while being able to make more of a difference, one patient at a time.

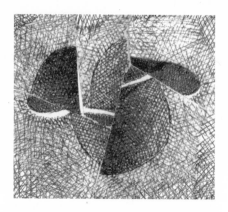

FIG. 5. *Hats 3.* Courtesy Tom Phillips and The Folio Society.

In her clinical role as a gerontology NP, Colleen has a broad sphere of influence because she is called upon by every clinical area in the hospital. She is able to generate questions about practice that she then takes through the research process, using the findings to implement changes that improve the quality of patient care. Her clinical and academic teaching opportunities also allow her to continually share with and learn from others. For example, in her story of a project that involved the surgical service — a project she described as "some really fun work" — Colleen emphasized the partnerships she works hard to develop:

We try really hard not to be the people that come and say,
"Oh we're from geriatrics and we know all about care for older
people, and we're going to tell you all the bad things that you do."
We really try to present it as a partnership with them because
they know all about their specialty and we know squat about it,
but we know about some of the issues that are happening and
the de-conditioning issues and these medication issues and all of
those things with the patients, so we're just trying to help put
this together.

Having observed that the surgeons had a high usage of "less senior-friendly medications," Colleen developed a partnership with a pharmacist in an attempt to alter the surgeons' prescribing patterns. Although she had been a colleague with the pharmacist for a long time, she noted that their relationship began to build in a different way when she became an NP. As a result of using one-on-one teaching opportunities combined with team presentations at surgical grand rounds, they were successful in eliminating the use of Tylenol #3 and Gravol, the two targeted medications, enabling her to affect patient care in additional ways.

Subsequent to this successful educational initiative, Colleen and the nursing manager for the orthopedics program engaged in a retrospective cost analysis for the targeted drugs before and after the teaching intervention period using the computerized medication records and discovered significant cost-savings. Colleen was eager to begin her next research project, which concerned Foley catheter usage and related nosocomial infection rates; this involved partnerships with some clinical nurses and a few student nurses. Colleen was replete with stories of how she made a difference by calling on all the competencies required in this advanced nursing practice role.

And then as an NP, when I'm doing consults, they'll ask me questions, whether it's the nurses on the team or the social workers in discharge planning. . . . When I first started as an NP we really wanted our team to try and develop a geriatric assessment form that was more interdisciplinary so that I wasn't going and doing a cognitive assessment and the occupational therapist was going and doing the same cognitive assessment. We wanted to make it with the understanding that it could be any of the team members contributing to that. So we worked on this and now we've taken it regionally and we're going to standardize it so that we are not repeating work across institutions and we're helping to build trust in each other as colleagues. *We also made a conscious choice to generate a problem list rather than the diagnosis list, which helps us to focus on the patient and their issues, and lets all the health care professionals create or add to the list. Now we need to work on the discharge planning based on the patient-centred list.*

The third story is told by Grace, an NP with the designated job title of NP/CNS who worked within a cardiology program. Being more for Grace is about the ability to influence change on many levels by being actively involved in all domains of practice. The advanced-practice NP role offers her the opportunity to "do everything." As a result, there are always new learning opportunities with new challenges "to mentally turn [her] on, to stimulate [her]." She is constantly stretched, but then observes ripple effects not only on patient care, but also on the nursing staff and even on the physicians. Being more is about "the whole package of advanced practice" and, as such, is "just the perfect nursing role."

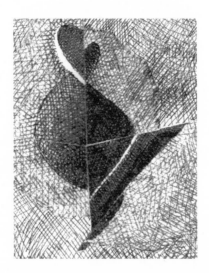

FIG. 6. *Hats 4.* Courtesy Tom Phillips and The Folio Society.

Grace's practice is built on a belief "that most nurses have the knowledge to do a lot of things that NPs do; they can do a lot of things physicians do, but what prevents them is that the structure doesn't allow them to practise to that level." Therefore, she sees the NP role as a first step to expanding the role of the staff nurse. The reader might recall Grace's story about learning to remove arterial sheaths after cardiac catheterization as described in chapter 3. Grace later recounted the evolution of the performance of this procedure. Once she became confident and comfortable removing arterial sheaths and managing any related complications, Grace noted that the patients were required to remain flat in bed for six hours after sheath removal, although homeostasis at the site takes only thirty to forty-five minutes. Believing this practice was a "sacred cow," she initiated a randomized controlled trial that assigned patients to two, four, or six hours of bed rest and compared all vascular complications across the three groups.

I had physicians whose only conception of a nurse in research was the people who helped them with their research. Most of them in the group had never heard of a nurse being a principal investigator on a research study actually conducting independent research. . . . When I presented my research findings, every cardiologist in the department took time out of their schedule to come to my presentation and they all asked questions. And there were staff nurses who came in on their day off. Before I'd even started doing the research, I said, "I'm not going to go through all this as a paper exercise. If this shows that it's safe to reduce bed rest, then we need to implement the change." And we all agreed as an advisory group that we would implement that change. And the day after I presented the findings, the change of practice went into effect. We went from six hours to two hours, which is really cool. It was better for the patients and decreased the workload for the nurses.

At the time of the study's implementation, Grace noted that there was a large core of expert, experienced nurses who were interested in learning to do the procedure. Grace felt that seeing her manage sheath removal made it easier for them to say, "Well, if she can do it, I can do it too." Although she supported them, she requested they wait to lobby for the expansion of their practice until after the trial; she needed to hold constant the quality of sheath removal, so as not to bias the complication rates. In the interim, she encouraged them to be involved in the study and used this time to help them develop a proposal. The results of the study fuelled their enthusiasm, and they argued in the proposal that the time previously allocated to caring for patients on bed rest could now be allocated to the sheath removal procedure. Grace was physically present on the unit to support the nurses in the management of complications arising: "Occasionally, they'd pull the sheath and the groin clamp would come off and then the patient would re-bleed later. The experienced nurses would always put the groin clamp on and then call me and I'd come and say, 'Oh, it's fine. You've done a great job. Just carry on.'"

Recognizing that the dynamic of a change in nursing practice often rests with physicians, "because if the physicians aren't convinced that it's going to be safe then practice isn't going to change," Grace presented the research results and their program change at an international medical and nursing conference: "And so I had two very stats-related, safety-driven presentations for the medical audience and then two more patient-focused ones in the nursing sessions." As a result of disseminating the findings at the conference, her colleagues in several hospitals across the country changed their practices. The ripple effects were exciting and personally satisfying:

The neat thing was not only changing practice on our unit but changing practice well outside that. And for a lot of physicians it was something completely new to them to realize that a nurse can do clinically relevant research that changes practice in a positive way. And it was wonderful to see the ripple effects of that on the staff. After that, when I was being introduced to the new staff on the floor by the senior staff, they introduced me as, "This is our nurse practitioner. She's the one who's responsible for all the bed rest research." So it was the research that they were focusing on. One staff member sought me out at a professional nursing meeting and said, "I've heard all about your research and I'd really love to work with you on nursing research." And he said "nursing research." But when they can see that they can actually use this stuff and be involved in it, it's great to see them turned on.

These three NPs' stories reveal that this search to be more through being an advanced practitioner is associated with a personal moral imperative of exercising their strengths in the context of close relationships within and outside their communities of practice in a transformative or empowering way. Rather than focusing on the obstacles to their progress, they deftly go over, under, and around them. They are not concerned with what nurses and others should or should not be doing; instead, they are concerned with how nurses and others can do anything they want and need to do. They are transforming their own and others' lives through their strengths and their intent to give others, particularly nurses, the tools to claim their strengths and use them to live their professional lives to the fullest. Thus, sharing and using power to strengthen others is a constitutive element of their role as advanced practitioners. NPs demonstrate this vividly when they make a public demonstration of recognition for the Other's perspective, thus validating, honouring, and valuing the Other's knowledge and skills. They challenge the power-over perspective by asking, "Why would you not include those who have the knowledge and skills? Why would you not hold those who do the job accountable for looking for the gaps, identifying redundancies, and knowing how to find the solutions? Why is there a need to tell bright people what to do? Why do we not work together to solve problems?" They know their own limitations — "I am not super-duper," "I am not a super nurse, because again that's not being respectful of my nursing colleagues. We are all there to provide patient care and we all bring something vital and important to the care of the patient" — but imagine the possibilities in others. In this way, NPs identify themselves as nurses without any extraordinary power and work hard to help others find the power within. As a result, paradoxically, their power is amplified, as is their sense of the possible. They may be inspired to say as Morpheus does to Neo in the movie *The Matrix* (1999): "I'm going to show you a world without borders or boundaries — a world where anything is possible."

Driven by a desire to always be more challenged and more connected with the nursing profession, NPs in being advanced practitioners continuously expand their communities of practice through multiple and varied partnerships. They strive to make more visible for nurses and others that which has heretofore been invisible and silent, and they work hard to involve others, particularly staff nurses, in every element of what they do. At this point in their journey, having the opportunity to be pioneers means that they can lead the process of creating a vision, the final appearance of which no one really knows, the diversity of which is limited only by their own imaginations and the imaginations of others. From this perspective, NPs acknowledge that the results are out of their hands, since they are involved in a mutual process they even invite and encourage. However, they are open to the options available and involve themselves in creating the changes they intend without having an attachment to the outcomes. Barrett (2010) would refer to this way of engaging in the world as *power*, defined as knowing participation in change, and as such she would likely see these NPs as living *power-as-freedom*, leading the change process from the perspective that power is inclusive and unlimited, with outcomes frequently not predetermined. Being an advanced practitioner enables NPs to achieve levels of scale and complexity that give new dimensions to their belonging. Interestingly, the Old French word *pio(u)ner* carried the meanings "dig," "excavate," and "mine." And pioneering NPs in fact unearth rich stores and abundant rewards inherent in being advanced practitioners. They find a greater sense of personal fulfillment as nurses through their opportunities to make a more diverse and broader difference to their patients, families, and the nursing profession, and they discover more of their own possibilities for being who they desire to be. Barrett (2010, p. 47) might describe NPs, in being advanced practitioners, as "quiet rebel[s] with a pioneering spirit," a perspective that sees the pioneering journey continue to this day and beyond.

These last three NPs' stories reveal that in being advanced practitioners, NPs do more than participate in each of the practice competencies. They engage in building and nurturing communities of practice that have the patient and families as the core focus, and they develop partnerships that foster the growth and development of others, particularly (but not only) nurses, to make the best delivery of care possible. They also conduct community-building conversations and negotiate new situations through partnerships in projects, research, and teaching centred on patient-care issues. Through their ongoing development of interpersonal relationships, they pursue common enterprises in concert with nurses, physicians, dieticians, pharmacists, social workers, and others. As a result of engaging in shared activities, they create a history of shared experiences. Through their efforts, they build and expand the level of competence within their communities of practice, through these interacting trajectories. Consequently, their identities and those of others are continually being shaped in relationship to one another. As advanced practitioners, they expand the boundaries of nursing and open the peripheries to allow for engagement with all those who work within these communities.

These stories also reveal that NPs' imaginations come from a place of stepping back and looking at their engagement "through the eyes of an outsider" (Wenger, 1998, p. 185). By reflecting on others' experiences, they imagine the possibilities in the situation and in others; they see themselves in new ways and imagine the "multiple constellations" (p. 185) that could be contexts for their practices. They explore other ways of doing what they do, take risks, and create unlikely connections. In fact, there is some degree of "playfulness" (p. 185) in how they engage in their work. As several NPs observed, they are having fun in discovering being more. Moreover, they are able to make visible and bring voice to what they do through the day-to-day sharing of their stories and explanations. By involving others in the processes of research, project work, writing, presenting, and problem-solving, those others, like them, begin to imagine "the present as only one of many possibilities and the future as a number of possibilities" (p. 185).

Perhaps as a result of reaching out to their colleagues in understanding, NPs as advanced practitioners begin to feel understood (Dickson, 1991). Through reverent attention to nurturing engagements with their communities of practice, NPs create an opening and emerge with the perception of being transformed. As Nichols (2005, p. 10) noted, there is a strong connection between "reverent attention to nurturing engagements" and "feeling understood" that strengthens the sense of belonging and sense of self:

> If listening strengthens our relationships by cementing our connection with another, it also fortifies our sense of self. In the presence of a receptive listener, we're able to

clarify what we think and discover what we feel. Thus, in giving an account of our experience to someone who listens, we are better able to listen to ourselves. Our lives are co-authored in dialogue.

This way of engaging may be similar to what Reay and colleagues (Reay, Golden-Biddle, and GermAnn, 2006) referred to as "cultivating opportunities grounded in NPs' embeddedness." While embeddedness serves to constrain some NPs, it may also facilitate action because it serves as a "means of stratification by opening windows of opportunity" (Dacin, Ventresca, and Beal, 1999, p. 335). NPs use their embeddedness, or engagement with others in their community of practice, as a source of opportunity "to evaluate the potential success of specific strategies and choose particular times and places to act" (Reay, Golden-Biddle, and GermAnn, 2006, p. 979). In being advanced practitioners, NPs continue to develop and apply their deep knowledge of the system and its actors in order to select and frame arguments for making changes within clinical practice, and they use their understanding of their communities to recognize and take advantage of opportunities.

Now, NPs subtly remove system barriers and prove the value of the NP role in richer and deeper ways (Reay, Golden-Biddle, and GermAnn, 2006). In being advanced practitioners, they find they can make more of a difference and "secure small wins" (p. 990), working at the front line day by day and interaction by interaction. Gradually they are seen by others as being more. Paradoxically, in finding ways to fit the NP role into already established systems and structures, they also change the system to accommodate this new role and in doing so find the perfect fit for themselves. Once they create and strengthen their connections in new ways, they begin to recognize that the NP role will be relatively difficult to disconnect or eliminate.

Administration sees the ripple effect on patient care, the staff, and even the physicians. I mean, some practices have changed for the better because of the research we do on questions that arise from our own practice. Nurses feel better informed. We hear that the patients are happy with the care we provide. I think they know that they would lose a great deal if they got rid of this role now.

These NPs' stories illuminate a life in a process of a multiplicity of assemblages, of connections, and of interactions. In being more as advanced practitioners, NPs are not attached to an official structure, a rigid pattern, or an imposed or straightforward stream of thought. They engage in what perhaps could be thought of as "rhizomatic thought" (Holmes and Gastaldo, 2004, p. 261) — that is, their lives emerge and grow in simultaneous, multiple ways, without a beginning or an ending, and are in a constant state of play, a process that may be fostered because they are pioneers. In this way, NPs become capable of promoting the creation of new concepts that allow for the emergence of alternative possibilities for themselves, others, and nursing. They demonstrate an ability to tolerate ambiguity and chaos, and do not rely on certitudes to progress or develop new ways of being for themselves or nursing. Their imaginations allow them to continuously become Other, and they are willing to take the risks and face the challenges associated with the metamorphosis. In this way of living their work, they discover being more and find the perfect fit.

A transmuting sea star
Caught on a watery coil
In uncharted waters.

— Mika Yoshimoto (2008, x)

Chapter 6

Breaking Silence and Giving Voice

It is not easy to be a pioneer — but oh, it is fascinating!
I would not trade one moment, even the worst moment,
for all the riches in the world.
— Elizabeth Blackwell, *Pioneer Work in Opening the Medical
Profession to Women: Autobiographical Sketches*
(quoted in Grant and Carter, 2004, p. 11)

How does one end that which is only the beginning? This work
began with the question *What is the experience of acute-care* NPs? In
seeking to answer it, I have considered the influences that have
shaped my own perception of NP practice and the ways in which
they are understood in our society. I have tried to create a description of their transformational journey as the NP experiences it

❖ 257 ❖

and to evoke some of its essential aspects. Through deepening our understanding of the nature of their nursing practice, this work serves to make visible aspects of the NP role as lived that have heretofore been invisible. This way of knowing and understanding NPs makes it possible for NPs to use a different voice in professional and social discourse, and for health care providers and health care recipients to enter the conversation in new and diverse ways; we can break the silence on who the NP is and how NP nursing practice unfolds in all its uniqueness and complexity.

The NPs' transformational journey of being and becoming in this role is an attempt to create a context in which to proceed with their professional lives. The journey involves, among other things, being competent, confident, and comfortable with the clinical management of their patients; having fun, doing well, feeling good about what they are able to accomplish and how it is accomplished; dealing with boredom; thinking about the future; and struggling to maintain a sense of self they feel they can live with. Their journey is about finding the perfect fit, the experience of which occurs through their engagement in practice. In this sense, it is not only about navigating a way into the future, but also involves being called to draw upon the past.

At this time in Canadian nursing history, the nature of being NPs in acute-care settings is as much about writing a history as it is about drawing a map. Yet, paradoxically in some respects, this must be an uncharted journey, for the experience of being an NP within this context takes its own shape for each person. It is not as if nurses who choose to become NPs all set sail from the same port and then reach a fixed destination, via a predetermined route, using the same compass within a designated timeframe. Their journeys come into existence moment by moment as they are lived within their communities of practice. NPs' daily practices, with their mixture of submission and assertion, are complex, collectively negotiated responses to what they understand their situation to be (Wenger, 1998, p. 78). Their journeys are not reducible to a single element such as power, satisfaction, competition, collaboration, desire, or economic relations. Just as Wenger discovered in his work on communities of practice, how NPs go about doing their work and who they are is a complex mixture of power and dependence, expertise and helplessness, success and failure, alliance and competition, ease and struggle, authority and collegiality, resistance and compliance, fun and boredom, trust and suspicion.

There is a shift in NPs' relationships within each of their communities of practice throughout the journey. This shift occurs in a subtle and complex fashion. Yet all the while, the change gradually uncovers the differences between the NP and traditional clinical nursing roles, and between the NP and physician roles to which they are also somewhat similar. Every newly constructed difference in how work is conducted as a result of their presence, every new negotiation between physician and NP or bedside nurse and NP, as well as every new merger of work activities brought from the nursing and medical worlds, brings about a change in both the ecology of the communities of practice and the NP's sense of self in this role. As a result, NPs begin to see themselves anew and gradually undergo an inner transformation. In addition, others, particularly nurses, have the opportunity to see nursing in a new way, as well as new possibilities for being.

The question that guided this work was intended to allow the phenomenon to show itself. The paradoxical nature of hermeneutic phenomenological inquiry is that while there is a deeper and richer understanding of the question, something of itself must be held in reserve. The very thing that aims to uncover what is hiding is that which restricts it (Moules, 2002). Instead, the power of this work is found in its ability to have the question live on, seeking never to be complete, just more deeply and richly understood. The aim was to describe and find meaning in the NPs' lived experience; to that end, the intended aim has been accomplished. However, in Moules' terms, this inquiry is a "work in progress," and thus, in the truest sense, remains unfinished.

However, this understanding does not mean that there is not a response to the recognition that occurs when something rings true of what is said in the particular. Max van Manen (2002, p. 88) asserted that understanding in the phenomenological sense has the potential to sponsor more "thoughtful action: action full of thought and thought full of action." In other words, possibilities for different ways of understanding and being with NPs in education, practice, or research are planted and cultivated as a result of bringing forth something new or recognizing that which has been taken for granted. How may we attend to the conversation in a helpful way and move it beyond the singular voice of instrumentation and economics? How may we support the development of nurses as NPs as they undertake their journey? How may we help them be safe without diminishing the vulnerability and openness necessary for meaningful growth and transformation? How do we create dwellings of boundless possibilities for NPs in the acute-care context? Perhaps we should consider these questions from Heidegger's definition of dwelling (quoted in Devall and Sessions, 1985, pp. 98–99):

> Dwelling is not primarily inhabiting but taking care of and creating that space within which something comes into its own and flourishes. Dwelling is primarily saving, in the older sense of setting something free to become itself, what it essentially is. . . . Dwelling is that which cares for things so that they essentially presence and come into their own.

It is imperative to keep the questions open and expand the conversation. For example, given the new thoughts concerning how NPs are assigned various titles and the influence titles can have on the enactment and meaning of the role for the NP, we need to keep the discussion of titling in play at the local and national level. Title confusion and lack of role clarity continue to pose substantial barriers to NPs' full integration into acute-care settings across Canada. Donald and colleagues (2010, p. 203) recommended that to reduce confusion and facilitate communication, nursing regulators across the country should consider agreeing on common specialty titles. However, we also need to engage in a deeper and broader discussion that includes how titles, such as NP/CNS, NP, and CNS/NP, impact role clarity and the NP's identity of self.

This work has sought to humanize the NPs' experience as a transformational journey; now nurse educators and local administrators need to question what strategies best meet the changing needs of NPs through the various transitional processes they experience. Questions and ongoing engagement in intimate dialogue with NPs about what the perfect fit looks like for each person are essential in creating a dwelling of possibility. For instance, what supports are offered to the NPs in their institutions in terms of mentorship, not only in the clinical management of patients, but also in terms of the development of the research, leadership, and pedagogic acumen of individuals in the NP role? What are the teams' strategies for incorporating the NP role? How willing are the members of the community of practice to accept the NP role, and what are their understandings of this advanced nursing practice role? How can we create an environment that fosters imagination?

The visibility of the ways in which NPs make a difference — while embedded in a moral imperative of caring and as integrated with some of the traditional medical curing activities — raises questions concerning the structure of their practices. If the additional time spent with patients and their families is more conducive to holistic care — which is ultimately more healing for patients and more satisfying for NPs — should their practices be restructured in such a way to afford that time? At the very least, the possibility of NPs to transcend the binary opposition of care and cure, thus opening a new space for being, as has been revealed by them, should provoke the nursing profession to pause and reconsider the discourse that has asked "Whither the 'nurse' in nurse practitioner?" (Weston, 1975)

We need to acknowledge the NPs' experience. Explication of the nature of their journey also calls into question the tendency to underestimate the complexities of taking on this role. All of us, including educators, administrators, nurses at the bedside, and physicians, need to recognize and acknowledge the profound effect the transformational journey has on them. We also need to recognize and acknowledge that their journey does not end with the attainment of competence, confidence, and comfort in the direct patient-care competency. To dismiss this knowledge is to underestimate the power their experience has upon their identity, their sense of belonging, and how they embody their practice. Being disconnected, being uncertain, and being lost, for example, are experiences that NPs have held in silence, in the assumption that these are problems particular to the individual. How many NPs have left (or could leave) this role as a result of misunderstanding that these feelings are theirs alone? How can we use this information to lessen their feelings of isolation and help NPs to engage in a dialectic that will enhance the transformation from being adrift to being NPs?

Answers to such questions as: *Has anyone else felt like this?*, *What is happening to me?*, *Is this normal?*, and *How will I know when I am good enough?* — do not lie only in the findings of this study. On the contrary, every NP must undertake and learn from his or her own journey. Nevertheless, the NPs' transformational journey as revealed here is important, as a place from which they can perceive and understand their own experience. Initiating a dialogue with openness to who they are and who they want to be, with an appreciation of the journey, can promote self-discovery and development of the imagination.

The most important aspect of such questions may lie in the search for answers rather than in the answers themselves. Heidegger (1968) wrote in *What is Called Thinking?*, "And yet the question may even be such that it will never allow us to go through, but instead requires that we settle down and live within it" (p. 137). This may be true for questions about being and becoming an NP as well. All of us who work with NPs need to dwell within the questions. We, too, need to focus on the development of our imaginations regarding the possibilities for the NP role in acute-care settings and the ways in which we can foster NPs in their transformational journey.

Consider again the question: *How does one end that which is only the beginning?* "A man went to knock at the king's door and said, 'Give me a boat.'" So begins José Saramago's (1999, p. 1) simple but intriguing short story *The Tale of the Unknown Island*, a fable that carefully conveys the story of a transformational journey. An unnamed man arrives at the king's "door for petitions," a door the king neglects because he is waiting by the "door for favors," which are favours that others offer to him. Fortunately, the man's tenacity coincides with the ruler's fear of a popular revolt, which results in the king grudgingly granting the man a seaworthy boat with which he can sail to find "the unknown island." In the ensuing philosophical discussion about whether such an island could be found or even existed, it is revealed that the unknown man is a dreamer, with bold imagination and strong will. When the king assures him that all the islands have already been discovered, the man refuses to believe it, explaining that man exists "simply because there can't possibly not be an unknown island" (Saramago, 1999, p. 12). Having overheard the entire conversation, the palace cleaning woman leaves the royal residence to join the man on his voyage of discovery. The two would-be explorers claim the boat, only to realize they have no provisions, map, or crew. Whether the vessel ever finds its destination remains a mystery, but several crucial lessons endure: (1) Follow your dream and your dream will follow you; (2) If you don't step outside yourself, you'll never discover who you are; and (3) When sailing, there are more teachers along the way than you can ever expect or predict.

Some NPs find the perfect fit for which they are searching in being NPs. However, in being NPs they continue to live with the tension of being pulled to be more. It is unknown whether the tensions they experience will ever be experienced as an internal call to continue their journey. Melville informed us in *Moby Dick* that New Bedford at best is a point of departure, not a final destination, and only exists in relation to the journey out. As such, the journey out constitutes New Bedford as a temporary resting point, a way station, from which one begins another journey. Melville called on us to live "landless" and "shoreless," to continuously journey out from safe harbours upon a voyage that is open and for which there can be no final destination or end point. There are some NPs who continuously answer this call and are constantly challenging themselves to think about nursing and health care delivery in new ways, to leave the comfort and safety of what they think they know to be true about both, to imagine what could be, and to act and relate in new ways. It remains a mystery at this point where they will journey from here, but their journey is not over, because for NPs who live the experience of being more, being more is about the constant search for more. Some already imagine furthering their education in order to bring more knowledge and ideas to their practice, while others imagine a nursing practice that is more global. Perhaps for NPs who experience being more, their lived experience is similar to Geena Davis's belief, as quoted in Morris (1999, p. 320):

I view life as a journey. It's not so much having some goal and getting to it. It's taking the journey itself that matters. . . . I don't think life is about arriving somewhere and then just hanging out. It's expanding and expanding and trying and trying to get somewhere new and never stopping. It's getting out your colors and showing them.

This book concerns the experience of NPs as pioneers in Canada as they try to find a sense of identity while they negotiate Canadian sociocultural values concerning the way we traditionally deliver health care. The struggles that NPs experience often involve issues of estrangement from hegemonic values concerning nursing, medicine, and health care delivery in our society. It is my hope that this book inspires openness and dialogue between people within and across disciplines and the various health care sectors. I hope that the book's contents disrupt the current discourse that accommodates NPs only within the scope of its fixed values. I encourage other voices to come forth as well in order to share their stories, so that in breaking the silence, we can live within, converse about, and reflect upon this other side of silence.

[T]hat one most perilous and long voyage ended, only begins a second; and a second ended, only begins a third . . .
— **Herman Melville,** *Moby Dick*

References

Alcott, L.M. (1950). *Little women*. Garden City, New York: Nelson Doubleday.

Algase, D.L., & Whall, A.F. (1993). Rosemary Ellis' views on the substantive structure of nursing. *Image: Journal of Nursing Scholarship, 25*(1), 69-72.

Altrows, J. (2002). *Feeling like an imposter*. Retrieved from http://www. phenomenologyonline.com/sources/textorium/altrows-k-j-2002-feeling-like-an-imposter/

American Academy of Nurse Practitioners (2010). *Nurse practitioner cost effectiveness*. Retrieved from http://www.aanp.org/AANPCMS2/About AANP/QualityandCostEffectivenessOfNPCare.htm

Anderson, E.M., Leonard, B.J., & Yates, J.A. (1974). Epigenesis of the nurse practitioner role. *American Journal of Nursing, 74*(10), 1812-16.

Aoki, T. (2005). Imaginaries of "East and West": Slippery curricular signifiers in education. In W.F. Pinar & R.L. Irwin (Eds.), *Curriculum in a new key: The collected works of Ted. T. Aoki* (pp. 313-19). Mahwah, New Jersey: Lawrence Erlbaum Associates.

Baca, J.S. (1992). *Working in the dark: Reflections of a poet of the barrio*. Santa Fe, New Mexico: Red Crane Books.

Barer, M.L., & Stoddart, G.L. (1992a). Background, process, and perceived problems. *Canadian Medical Association Journal, 146*(3), 345-51.

Barer, M.L., & Stoddart, G.L. (1992b). Graduates of foreign medical schools. *Canadian Medical Association Journal, 146*(9), 1919-24.

Barer, M.L., & Stoddart, G.L. (1992c). Undergraduate medical training. *Canadian Medical Association Journal, 147*(3), 305-12.

Barnhart, R.K. (1988). *The Barnhart dictionary of etymology*. New York: H.W. Wilson.

Barrett, E.A.M. (2010). Power as knowing participation in change: What's new and what's next. *Nursing Science Quarterly, 23*(1), 47-54.

Bartlett, J., & Kaplan, J. (Eds.) (1992). *Bartlett's familiar quotations* (16th ed.). New York: Little, Brown and Company.

Bates, B. (1990). Twelve paradoxes: A message for nurse practitioners. *Journal of the American Academy of Nurse Practitioners, 2*(4), 136-39.

Beal, J.A., & Quinn, M. (2002). The nurse practitioner role in the NICU as perceived by parents. *The American Journal of Maternal Child Nursing, 27*(3), 183-88.

Beckett, P. (2009). *Luminality*. Retrieved from http://beckettart.blogspot.com/ 2009/07/luminality.html

Beckett, S. (1955). *Waiting for Godot*. London: The Folio Society.

Benner, P. (1984). *From novice to expert*. Menlo Park, California: Addison-Wesley Publishing.

Benner, P. (1994). The tradition and skill of interpretive phenomenology in studying health, illness, and caring practices. In P. Benner (Ed.), *Interpretive phenomenology: Embodiment, caring, and ethics in health and illness* (pp. 99-127). Thousand Oaks, California: Sage.

Benner, P., Hooper-Kyriakidis, P., & Stannard, D. (1999). *Clinical wisdom and intervention in critical care: A thinking-in-action approach.* Philadelphia: W.B. Saunders.

Benner, P., Tanner, C., & Chesla, C. (1996). *Expertise in nursing practice: Caring, clinical judgment, and ethics.* New York: Springer.

Bergum, V. (2003). Relational pedagogy. Embodiment, improvisation, and interdependence. *Nursing Philosophy, 4*(2), 121–128.

Bergum, V., & Dosseter, J. (2003). *Relational ethics: The full meaning of respect.* Hagerstown, MD: University Publishing Group.

Bishop, A.H., & Scudder, J.R. (1990). *The practical, moral, and personal sense of nursing: A phenomenological philosophy of practice.* Albany, New York: State University of New York Press.

Boudreau, T. (1972). *Report of the Committee on Nurse Practitioners.* Ottawa, Ontario: Health and Welfare Canada.

Bowker, G.C., Timmermans, S., & Star, S.L. (1995). Infrastructure and organizational transformation: Classifying nurses' work. In W. Orlikowski, G. Walsham, M. Jones, & J. DeGross (Eds.), *Information technology and changes in organizational work* (pp. 244–370). London, England: Chapman and Hall.

Boykin, A., & Schoenhofer, S. (2001). *Nursing as caring: A model for transforming practice.* New York: Jones & Bartlett, National League for Nursing Press.

Brown, M.A., & Draye, M.A. (2003). Experiences of pioneer nurse practitioners in establishing advanced practice roles. *Journal of Nursing Scholarship, 35*(4), 391–97.

Bryant-Lukosius, D., Green, E., Fitch, M., Macartney, G., Robb-Blenderman, L., McFarlane, S., …Milne, H. (2007). A survey of oncology advanced practice nurses in Ontario: Profile and predictors of job satisfaction. *Canadian Journal of Nursing Leadership, 20*(2), 51–69.

Brykczynski, K.A. (1985). *Exploring the clinical practice of nurse practitioners.* (Unpublished doctoral dissertation.) University of California.

Brykczynski, K.A., & Lewis, P.H. (1997). Interpretive research exploring the healing practices of nurse practitioners. In P. Kritek (Ed.), *Reflections on healing: A central nursing construct* (pp. 518–34). New York: National League of Nursing Press.

Buehler, J. (1987). *Nurses and physicians in transition.* Ann Arbor, Michigan: UMI Research Press.

Buytendijk, F.J.J. (1961). *Pain.* (E. O'Sheil, Trans.). Westport, Connecticut: Greenwood Press.

Canadian Institute of Health Information (CIHI). (2006). *The regulation and supply of nurse practitioners in Canada.* Retrieved from http://www.cihi.ca.

Canadian Institute of Health Information (CIHI). (2010). *Regulated nurses: Canadian trends, 2004 to 2008, Updated February 2010.* Ottawa, Ontario: Canadian Institute for Health Information. Retrieved from http://secure.cihi.ca/cihiweb/products/regulated_nurses_2004_2008_en.pdf.

Canadian Nurses Association (CNA). (2002). *Cost-effectiveness of the nurse practitioner role*. Ottawa, Ontario: Canadian Nurses Association.

Canadian Nurses Association (CNA). (2006). Report of 2005 dialogue on advanced nursing practice. Ottawa, Ontario: Canadian Nurses Association. Retrieved from http://www.cna-nurses.ca/CNA/ documents/pdf/publications/Report_2005_ANP_Dialogue_e.pdf.

Canadian Nurses Association (CNA). (2008). *Advanced nursing practice: A national framework*. Ottawa, Ontario: Canadian Nurses Association.

Canadian Nurses Association (CNA). (2009). Position statement: The nurse practitioner. Ottawa, Ontario: Canadian Nurses Association. November. Retrieved from http://www.cna-nurses.ca/CNA/documents/pdf/ publications/PS_Nurse_Practitioner_e.pdf.

Canadian Nurse Practitioner Initiative (CNPI). (2004). *Practice component literature review report: Advanced nursing practice and the primary health care nurse practitioner—Title, scope, and role*. December. Ottawa, Ontario: Canadian Nurses Association.

Canadian Nurse Practitioner Initiative (CNPI). (2005). *Education component: Literature review report*. February. Ottawa, Ontario: Canadian Nurses Association.

Carnegie, D. (1964). *How to win friends and influence people*. New York: Simon & Schuster. (Original work published 1936.)

Carnevale, F. (2001). How do you know what you know? An epistemological analysis of diagnostic reasoning in medicine. (Research report). Teaching Scholars Program, Faculty of Medicine, McGill University, Montreal, Quebec.

Carroll, L. (1865) 1971. *Alice's adventures in Wonderland* and *Through the looking-glass*, xxv. New York: Oxford University Press.

Carter, A. J. E., & Chochinov, A. H. (2007). A systematic review of the impact of the nurse practitioners on cost, quality of care, satisfaction and wait times in the emergency department. *Canadian Journal of Emergency Medicine, 9*(4), 286-95.

Cassell, J. (1992). On control, certitude, and the "paranoia" of surgeons. In J. Morse (Ed.), *Qualitative Health Research* (pp. 170-91). Thousand Oaks, California: Sage.

Centre for Nursing Studies (2001). *Final report: The nature of the extended/ expanded nursing role in Canada* (No. NA 321). Retrieved from http:// www.cns.nf.ca/research/finalreport.htm.

Cohen, M. H. (1995). The triggers of heightened parental uncertainty in chronic, life-threatening childhood illness. *Qualitative Health Research, 5*(1), 63-77.

Colquhoun, G. (2002). *Playing God: Poems about medicine*. Wellington: Steele Roberts Ltd.

Crane, S. (2003). *Aidan's way: The story of a boy's life and a father's journey*. Naperville: Sourcebooks.

Cummings, G. G., Fraser, K., & Tarlier, D. S. (2003). Implementing advanced nurse practitioner roles in acute care: An evaluation of organizational change. *Journal of Nursing Administration, 33*(3), 139-45.

Dacin, M. T., Ventresca, M. J., & Beal, P. D. (1999). The embeddedness of organizations: Dialogue and directions. *Journal of Management, 25*(3), 317-56.

D'Amour, D., Morin, D., Dubois, C., Lavoie-Tremblay, M., Dallaire, C., & Cyr, G. (2007). Évaluation de l'implantation du programme d'intéressement au titre d'infirmière praticienne spécialisée. Montréal, PQ: Centre Ferasi. Retrieved from http://www.ferasi.umontreal.ca/fra/0 7_info/Rapport% 20MSSS%20%20IPS.pdf.

Dana, R. H. (2001). *Two years before the mast.* New York: Random House. (Original work published 1840.)

Davidhizar, R. (1991). Ten strategies for increasing your self-confidence. *Journal of NSNA/Imprint,* (September/October), 105-8.

Devall, B., & Sessions, G. (1985). *Deep ecology.* Salt Lake City: Peregrine Books.

Dickson, M. P. (1991). Feeling understood: A heuristic research investigation (Unpublished doctoral dissertation). Villanova, PA: Villanova University.

Donald, F., Bryant-Lukosius, D., Martin-Misener, R., Kaasalainen, S., Kilpatrick, K., Carter, N., …DiCenso, A. (2010). Clinical nurse specialists and nurse practitioners: Title confusion and lack of role clarity. *Canadian Journal of Nursing Leadership, 23*(Special Issue), 189-210.

Dowie, J., & Elstein, A. (Eds.) (1988). *Professional judgement: A reader in clinical decision making.* Cambridge, MA: Cambridge University Press.

Dreyfus, H. L. (1992). Heidegger's history of the being of equipment. In H. L. Dreyfus & H. Hall (Eds.), *Heidegger: A critical reader* (pp. 173-85). Cambridge, MA: Blackwell.

Dreyfus, H. L. (1993). Heidegger on the connection between nihilism, art, technology, and politics. In C. Guignon (Ed.), *The Cambridge companion to Heidegger* (pp. 289-316). New York: Cambridge University Press.

Eliot, G. (2002). *Middlemarch.* New York: Random House. (Original work published 1871.)

Fadiman, A. (1997). *The spirit catches you and you fall down: A Hmong child, her American doctors, and the collision of two cultures.* New York: Farrar, Straus, & Giroux.

Fanta, K., Cook, B., Falcone, Jr., R., Rickets, C., Schweer, L., Brown, R., & Garcia, V. (2006). Pediatric trauma nurse practitioners provide excellent care with superior patient satisfaction for injured children. *Journal of Pediatric Surgery, 41*(1), 277-81.

Ferguson, F. (1991). Awaiting the diagnosis. *Phenomenology + Pedagogy, 9,* 312-18.

Fisher, S. (1995). *Nursing wounds: Nurse practitioners, doctors, women patients and the negotiation of meaning.* New Brunswick: Rutgers University Press.

Foucault, M. (1980). Power/knowledge: Selected interviews and other writings 1972-1977. New York: Pantheon.

Foucault, M. (1994). *The birth of the clinic: An archaeology of medical perception.* (A.M. Sheridan, Trans.). New York: Random House. (Original work published 1963.)

Frank, A. W. (1991). *At the will of the body.* New York: Houghton Mifflin.

Frank, A. W. (1995). *The wounded storyteller: Body, illness, and ethics.* Chicago: University of Chicago Press.

Frank, A. W. (2004). *The renewal of generosity: Illness, medicine, and how to live.* Chicago: University of Chicago Press.

Froggatt, K. (1997). Rites of passage and the hospice culture. *Mortality, 2*(2), 123–36.

Gadamer, H. G. (1989). *Truth and method* (2nd rev. ed.). (J. Weinsheimer & D. G. Marshall, Trans.). New York: Crossroad Publishing Company.

Gadow, S. (1980). Existential advocacy: Philosophical foundations of nursing. In S. F. Spicker & S. Gadow (Eds.), *Nursing–Images and ideals: Opening a dialogue with the humanities* (pp. 79–101). New York: Springer.

Gadow, S. (1989). Clinical subjectivity: Advocacy with silent patients. *Nursing Clinics of North America, 24*(2), 535–41.

Gadow, S. (1994). Whose body? Whose story? The question about narrative in women's health care. *Soundings, An Interdisciplinary Journal, 77*(3–4), 295–307.

Gordon, S. (2005). *Nursing against the odds: How health care cost cutting, media stereotypes, and medical hubris undermine nurses and patient care.* Ithaca, NY: Cornell University Press.

Gortner, S. R. (1982). Commentary. In, L. H. Aitken (Ed.), *Nursing in the 1980s: Crises, opportunities, challenges* (pp. 495–502). Philadelphia: Lippincott.

Grant, T., & Carter, S. (2004). *Women in medicine.* Richmond Hill: Firefly Books.

Haas, J., & Shaffir, W. (1987). *Becoming doctors: The adoption of a cloak of competence.* Greenwich: JAI Press.

Hall, S. (1990). Cultural identity and diaspora. In J. Rutherford (Ed.), *Identity: Community, culture and difference* (pp. 222–37). London: Lawrence & Wishart.

Hamilton, E. (1940). *Mythology: Timeless tales of gods and heroes.* Boston, Massachusetts: Little Brown & Co.

Hamric, A. B., Spross, J. A., & Hanson, C. M. (Eds.) (1996). *Advanced practice nursing: An integrative approach.* New York: Saunders Elsevier.

Harding, S. (1980). Value-laden technologies and the politics of nursing. In S. F. Spicker & S. Gadow (Eds.), *Nursing: Images and ideals* (pp. 49–75). New York: Springer.

Hawley, M. P. (2005). Making a difference in critical care nursing practice: An interpretive inquiry (Unpublished doctoral dissertation). University of Alberta, Edmonton.

Health Professions Regulatory Advisory Council (HPRAC). (2007a). *Scope of practice for registered nurses in the extended class (nurse practitioners): A jurisdictional review.* Toronto, ON: Health Professions Regulatory Advisory Council. Retrieved from http://www.hprac.org/en/projects/resources/hprac-nursing.jurisdictionalreview.november2007.final.pdf.

Health Professions Regulatory Advisory Council (HPRAC). (2007b). *Scope of practice for registered nurses in the extended class (nurse practitioners): A jurisdictional review, Appendix A.* Toronto, ON: Health Professions Regulatory Advisory Council. Retrieved from http://www.hprac.org/en/projects/resources/hprac-APPENDIXA-newcoverandindex.nov0507.pdf.

Hegel, G.W.F. (1971). *Hegel's philosophy of mind* (W. Wallace, Trans.). Oxford, UK: Clarendon Press. (Original translation published 1894.)

Heidegger, M. (1962). *Being and time* (J. Macquarrie & E. Robinson, Trans.). Oxford: Blackwell. (Original work published 1927)

Heidegger, M. (1966). Memorial address. (J.M. Anderson & E.H. Freund, Trans.). In *Discourse on thinking* (pp. 43-57). New York: Harper & Row. (Original work published 1959.)

Heidegger, M. (1968). *What is called thinking?* (J.G. Gray, Trans.). New York: Harper & Row. (Original work published 1954.)

Heidegger, M. (1971). Building, dwelling, thinking (A. Hofstadter, Trans.). In D.F. Krell (Ed.), *Basic writings: From being and time (1927) to* The task of thinking *(1964)* (2nd ed.) (pp. 347-63). New York: HarperCollins.

Heidegger, M. (1977). *The question concerning technology, and other essays* (W. Lovitt, Trans.). New York: Harper & Row. (Original work published 1954.)

Heitz, L., Steiner, S., & Burman, M. (2004). RN to FNP: A qualitative study of role transition. *Journal of Nursing Education, 43,* 416-21.

Hoffman, L.A., Tasota, F.J., Zullo, T.G., Scharfenberg, C., & Donahoe, M.P. (2005). Outcomes of care managed by an acute care nurse practitioner/attending physician team in a subacute medical intensive care unit. *American Journal of Critical Care, 14,* 121-32.

Holmes, D., & Gastaldo, D. (2004). Rhizomatic thought in nursing: An alternative path for the development of the discipline. *Nursing Philosophy, 5,* 258-67.

Hravnak, M., Kleinpell, R.M., Madgic, K.S., & Guttendorf, J. (2009). The acute care nurse practitioner. In A.B. Hamric, J.A. Spross, & C.M. Hanson (Eds.), *Advanced practice nursing: An integrative approach* (4th ed.) (pp. 403-36). St. Louis: Saunders/Elsevier.

Hurlock-Chorostecki, C., van Soreren, M., & Goodwin, S. (2008). The acute care nurse practitioner in Ontario: A workforce study. *Canadian Journal of Nursing Leadership, 21*(4), 100-116.

Jardine, D.W. (1998). *To dwell with a boundless heart.* New York: Peter Lang.

Johnson, J.L. (1994). A dialectical examination of nursing art. *Advances in Nursing Science, 17*(1), 1-14.

Kaasalainen, S., Martin-Misener, R., Kilpatrick, K., Harbman, P., Bryant-Lukosius, D., Donald, ...DiCenso, A. (2010). A historical overview of the development of advanced practice nursing roles in Canada. *Canadian Journal of Nursing Leadership, 23*(Special Issue), 35-60.

Katz, J. (1984). *The silent world of doctor and patient.* New York: Free Press.

Kelly, N.R., & Mathews, M. (2001). The transition to first position as nurse practitioner. *Journal of Nursing Education, 40*(4), 156-62.

Kilpatrick, K., Harbman, P., Carter, N., Martin-Misener, R., Bryant-Lukosius, D., Donald, F., ...DiCenso, A. (2010). The acute care nurse practitioner role in Canada. *Canadian Journal of Nursing Leadership, 23*(Special Issue), 114–38.

Kim, H. S. (1999). Critical reflective inquiry for knowledge development in nursing practice. *Journal of Advanced Nursing, 29*(5), 1205–12.

Kleinpell, R.M. (2002). The acute care nurse practitioner: An expanding opportunity for critical care nurses. *Critical Care Nurse, February* (Suppl.), 12–16, 74.

Kleinpell, R.M. (2005). Acute care nurse practitioner practice: Results of a 5-year longitudinal study. *American Journal of Critical Care, 14*, 211–21.

Kleinpell, R.M., Hravnak, M., Werner, K. E., & Guzman, A. (2006). Skills taught in acute care NP programs: A national survey. *The Nurse Practitioner, 31*, 7–13.

Kolcaba, K. (2003). *Comfort theory and practice.* New York: Springer Properties.

Kundera, M. (1984). *The unbearable lightness of being* (M.H. Heim, Trans.). New York: Harper & Row.

Leder, D. (1990). *The absent body.* Chicago: University of Chicago Press.

Leder, D. (1992). A tale of two bodies: the Cartesian corpse and the lived body. In D. Leder (Ed.), *The body in medical thought and practice* (pp. 17–35). Dordrecht: Kluwer Academic Publishers.

Levinas, E. (1996). Ethics as first philosophy. In R. Kearney & M. Rainwater (Eds.), *The Continental Philosophy Reader* (pp. 124–35). New York: Routledge.

Lewis, P. H., & Brykczynski, K. (1994). Practical knowledge and competencies of the healing role of the nurse practitioner. *Journal of the Academy of Nurse Practitioners, 6*(5), 207–13.

Locsin, R. C. (1995). Machine technologies and caring in nursing. *Image: Journal of Nursing Scholarship, 27*(3), 201–3.

Locsin, R. C. (1998). Technologic competence as caring in critical care. *Holistic Nursing Practice, 12*, 50–56.

Locsin, R. C. (2001). *Advancing technology, caring, and nursing.* Westport, CT: Auburn House.

Maalouf, A. (2000). *In the name of identity* (B. Bray, Trans.). New York: Penguin Group. (Original work published 1996.)

Marcel, G. (1948). *The philosophy of existence.* (Manya Harari, Trans.). London: Harvill Press.

Martel, Y. (2002). *Life of Pi.* Toronto: Vintage Canada.

Matthews, D. A., Suchman, A. L., & Branch, W. T. (1993). Making "connections": The therapeutic potential of patient–client relationships. *Annals of Internal Medicine, 118*, 973–77.

Melville, H. (1992). *Moby Dick.* New York: Penguin Books. (Original work published 1851.)

Merton, R., Reader, G. C., & Kendall, R. L. (Eds.) (1957). *The student physician.* Cambridge: Harvard University Press.

Meyer, S.C., & Miers, L.J. (2005). Cardiovascular surgeon and acute care nurse practitioner: Collaboration on postoperative outcomes. *AACN Clinical Issues, 16*(2), 149–58.

Mishler, E.G. (1984). *The discourse of medicine: Dialectics of medical interviews.* Norwood: Ablex.

Mitchell, G., & Santopinto, M. (1998). The expanded role nurse: A dissenting viewpoint. *Canadian Journal of Nursing Administration, 1*(4), 8–10, 14.

Mitchell-DiCenso, A., Guyatt, G., Marrin, M., Goeree, R., Willan, A., Southwell,…M., Baumann, A. (1996). A controlled trial of nurse practitioners in neonatal intensive care units. *Pediatrics, 98,* 1143–48.

Morris, T. (1999). *Philosophy for dummies.* Forest City: IDG Books Worldwide.

Moules, N.J. (2002). Hermeneutic inquiry: Paying heed to history and Hermes." *International Journal of Qualitative Methods, 1*(3), Article 1. Retrieved from http://ejournals.library.ualberta.ca/index.php/IJQM/index.

Nichols, M.P. (2005). *The lost art of listening.* New York: Guilford.

Nightingale, F. (1992). *Notes on nursing: What it is, and what it is not.* Philadelphia: Lippincott Raven. (Original work published 1859.)

Nurse Practitioners Association of Ontario (NPAO) (2005). *Primary health care nurse practitioner (PHC NP) Historical Perspective.* Retrieved from http://www.npao.org/history.aspx.

Office of Technology Assessment (1986). *Nurse practitioners, physician assistants, and certified nurse midwives: A policy analysis.* (Health Technology Case Study 37). Washington, DC: Office of Technology Assessment, U.S. Congress.

Offredy, M. (1998). The application of decision making concepts by nurse practitioners in general practice. *Journal of Advanced Nursing, 28*(5), 988–1000.

Paes, P., Mitchell, A., Hunsberger, M., Blatz, S., Watts, J., Dent,…Southwell, D. (1989). Medical staffing in Ontario neonatal intensive care units. *Canadian Medical Association Journal, 140*(11), 1321–6.

Patterson, C. (Ed.) (1997). *Visions and voices: The nurse practitioner today.* Troy: Newgrange Press.

Pérez-Reverte, A. (2001). *The nautical chart* (M.S. Peden, Trans.). New York: Harcourt.

Peschel, R.E., & Peschel, E.R. (1986). *When a doctor hates a patient and other chapters in a young physician's life.* Los Angeles: University of California Press.

Pinar W.F., & Irwin, R.L., (Eds.) (2005). *Curriculum in a new key: The collected works of Ted. T. Aoki.* Mahwah: Lawrence Erlbaum Associates.

Pringle, D. (2007). Nurse practitioner role: Nursing needs it. *Canadian Journal of Nursing Leadership, 20*(2), 1–5.

Proust, M. (1999). *The captive and the fugitive* (vol. 5), *In search of lost time* (C.K. Scott-Moncrieff & T. Kilmartin, Trans.). New York: Random House. (Original work published 1923.)

Purnell, M.J. (1998). Who really makes the bed? Uncovering technological dissonance in nursing. *Holistic Nursing Practice, 12,* 12–22.